Your
CANCER
Your
LIFE

Your CANCER Your LIFE

Dr Trish Reynolds
MBBS, FRACP

An OPTIMA book

First published in Australia in 1987 by
Greenhouse Publications Pty Ltd
This edition published in Great Britain in 1988 by
Macdonald Optima, a division of
Macdonald & Co. (Publishers) Ltd

A Pergamon Press plc company

British Library Cataloguing in Publication Data
Reynolds, Trish
    Your cancer, your life.
    1. Man. Cancer
    I. Title
    616.99′4

    ISBN 0-356-15417-3

Macdonald & Co. (Publishers) Ltd
3rd Floor
Greater London House
Hampstead Road
London NW1 7QX

Printed and bound in Great Britain by
The Guernsey Press Co. Ltd., Guernsey, Channel Islands.

CONTENTS

DEDICATION

To Debbie, Julie, Karen, Helen, Mary, Margaret and Wilhelminia. Through their refusal to be passive victims, they taught me a lot about living.

And to Megan and Viv, without whom I might not yet have explored and accepted my own strength.

ACKNOWLEDGEMENTS

My thanks to Barbara for her enthusiasm, skill and time.

INTRODUCTION

If you have picked up this book because you have cancer, you have just taken a very courageous step towards taking active control of your situation and away from being a passive victim. I write this book especially for you, a person living with cancer, and throughout it I will address you directly. But in my mind I also welcome many silent observers to our conversation and I'm sure you will too. You are not the only one for whom the information and perspectives of this book are important. They are also important for many people who don't have cancer.

Perhaps you have picked up this book because someone you love—a friend or family member—has cancer. Perhaps you fear cancer and hope to make your fear manageable by learning some facts. Perhaps you are a nurse, a social worker, a doctor, an occupational therapist, a physiotherapist, a pharmicist, a dietician, a chaplain or one of the many other people who come into contact with, or care for, people with cancer in the course of your work. Although I will not be addressing you directly, this book *is* for all of you.

For those of you who do have cancer, I know how frightening it is to seek out information. This takes a lot of courage, but I also know that it is well and truly worth the effort. Why? Because ignorance means helplessness and knowledge is power. In ignorance, your imagination may fill your body with a ghastly foreign monster which is devouring you, its helpless victim. With knowledge, you can work to accept realistically what you cannot change, while taking charge over every other aspect of your disease, treatment and lifestyle. With the right information you can make the best decisions for *you*. In ignorance, you must

1

passively accept recommendations from others. Knowing your rights as a patient, you can assert them.

You may have been seeing yourself as a tiny abandoned raft caught in a storm at sea. Waves crash over you, gales blow you where they will, you don't know where you are or where you are heading. No one is on board to make repairs or steer a course. The forces of the storm are gradually breaking you into pieces. At any moment you could be completely destroyed, torn apart by forces over which you have no control.

Try another picture. You are the captain of a huge modern ship in the same storm. Your powerful engines and sleek, low shape prevent the wind from blowing you off course. Although it is dark, you have all the instruments and power needed to keep you on course. You know exactly where you are. Waves crash over your ship but the steel hull is tough. Any damage is quickly repaired by the crew on board.

Both vessels are in terrifying situations.

Neither can be certain of survival.

Neither can control the storm.

But can't you *feel* the difference between the two? Sheer, numbing panic for the raft — no control over anything. Frightening on the ship, certainly, but feel how the terror is made manageable by taking responsibility — taking positive action and using available resources. Of course the ship could still go down in the storm, but never as a hopeless and helpless victim like the raft.

Which would you rather be — the abandoned raft bobbing at the mercy of the storm or the captain of the powerful ship? *The choice is yours.*

You can choose to be active, responsible and positive, to be in control of available resources rather than letting them control you. You can get information and guidance from doctors and other therapists, family, friends, books, magazines, films etc. Then, like the ship's captain, you can take the responsibility for making your own decisions. You have the right to be in charge of decisions such as who will treat you, what treatment you will have, where you will have it, for how long you will have it, who will have information about your medical condition, and so on.

2

It will sometimes seem easier to say: 'This is all too big and frightening for me. I don't want to know about it' or 'I couldn't possibly understand so I'd rather they didn't tell me anything' or 'The doctor is the expert and will always know what's best for me.' Fight the temptation. If you have these attitudes you will be like that abandoned raft with no control over your life.

Always keep this knowledge in the forefront of your mind: 'I am the greatest expert in the world on the topic of myself.' Your practitioner might know more than you about cancer, statistics, and possible treatments. Your family and friends might know more than you about their own needs and guess what they might do in your place. But *you* are the only one who knows how you feel and what is important for you, what price you are prepared to pay for possible recovery and when it is right for *you* to stop or refuse intensive treatment. You alone can combine this 'inside' unique personal knowledge with all the information you can get from the experts to make the best decisions for *you*.

If you want to be captain of the ship and not the raft, read this book. It will help you gain the information, and the confidence in your own rights and resources, that you need to be active and powerful in your battle with cancer.

Chapter 1

KNOW YOUR RIGHTS

The fact that you have cancer does not mean that you suddenly stop being an adult person with all the accepted and recognised rights of any adult person. It is *your* cancer, *your* body and *your* life. You are entitled to expect and get control over all important decisions to do with yourself. I have seen many patients give away their basic rights through ignorance, fear, awe, feelings of overwhelming helplessness and a need for protection. Unfortunately, giving away those rights completes a vicious circle—giving away rights leads to dependency on others, which leads to fear and helplessness, which leads to further giving away of rights and so on. You can break that vicious circle. Know about and insist on your rights to remain in control, that is, to function as a normal adult person, in every respect for which you remain physically and mentally able.

Let's be quite clear from the start just what you are up against. Most doctors and other practitioners who treat people with cancer want to be in complete control of the situation themselves. They are used to treating their patients like ignorant and dependent children. They are used, not to making recommendations, but to giving orders. They are used to their patients meekly and without question obeying those orders. Patients who do ask questions and want to make their own decisions are treated as a father might treat naughty, rebellious children. In an effort to eradicate what they see as a threat to their authority, they may act busy and important, patronise, cajole or intimidate.

So don't expect it to be easy. You are unlikely to get willing cooperation and may be treated with hostility, impatience, ridicule or condescension if you insist on clear explanations that will

5

enable you to make your own decisions. You must be prepared to deal with these tactics.

My main reason for writing this book is the knowledge that many, many people with cancer have suffered unnecessarily because they have left all the decisions to 'experts'. The aim of most cancer treatment 'experts' is *not* to make life as comfortable and pleasant as possible for their patients. Their main aim is to fight cancer and death. In this battle, the 'experts' often neglect to really care for the needs of those unique, whole, warm, individual people who happen to have cancer—like you.

Life is not going to be easy for you, now that you have cancer. Leaving the decisions to the 'experts' may mean that the rest of your life will be much less pleasant than it could have been. Making them yourself will be difficult, but will ensure that the decisions that are *best for you as a person* will be made.

I will discuss your rights under the following headings:
- Right to information, including:
  — right to have questions answered
  — right to as much time as necessary
  — right to more than one opinion.
- Right to control access to personal information.
- Right to make your own decisions.
- Rights in regard to research.
- Right to treatment by experienced practitioners.
- Right to care of your whole self.

RIGHT TO INFORMATION

You may initially feel very apprehensive about insisting on this. Let me tell you from my experience with many patients that your imagination will usually paint a far gloomier picture than the truth. It is much easier to grapple with facts than with the unknown. It is impossible to make good decisions in a black cloud of ignorance. These are very good reasons for insisting on the facts.

I know that some of you will be seeking information, advice and treatment from people other than medical-school trained doctors. I wish to make it clear that my training was as a medical doctor. I worked in a large teaching hospital. This is where my experience lies and it is what I understand best. Because of this, you will find that all the detailed explanations in this book concern the methods of diagnosis, assessment and treatment used by medical practitioners. In these sections I will use the word doctor to mean medical-school trained doctors. Some sections of this book, including all of this chapter, apply whether or not the cancer 'expert' you are consulting is a doctor. In these sections I will use the word 'practitioner' to mean whoever is looking after you, whatever their training.

Right to have Questions Answered

Before deciding on the best course of action you need answers to all of these questions:
- Do I have cancer?
- What is cancer and how does it spread?
- What is the name of my particular type of cancer?
- How was/can the diagnosis be made?
- Is it absolutely certain?
- Which parts of my body are affected?
- What tests are recommended?
- What would these tests involve?
- What would be the reasons for doing them?
- What are the results of the tests I have had and what does this mean for me?
- Is it possible to completely cure my cancer?
- What treatments are possible?
- What treatment does my practitioner recommend and why?
- What is the aim of each possible treatment?
  (To cure the cancer, temporarily control it, or control its symptoms?)
- What will happen if I have no actual anti-cancer treatment?
- What is the chance of achieving the aim of each treatment?

- If the aim is for temporary control, how long is this likely to last?
- How long before I will know whether my treatment is achieving its aim?
- How do I tell?
- How long, on average, do people like me live with each possible treatment?
- Exactly how is each possible treatment alternative administered?
- What are the likely unpleasant side effects of treatment?
- Can they be prevented or controlled and how?
- Are they temporary or permanent?
- How is each treatment likely to influence my lifestyle (time in hospital, in bed, off work, etc)?

Remember that, because every patient is different, and because no one can look with certainty into the future, many of the answers can only be educated guesses—what is average or likely. No one can tell you exactly how *you* will react to a certain treatment or how long *you* will live. The best anyone can do is tell you what is *likely* to happen. It is important to know this, and also to know what could happen if you are *not* an 'average' patient, that is both the best and worst that *could* happen.

Remember you cannot make the best decisions for yourself without this information. Getting it will not be easy. Most of the answers should come from your practitioner. You can ask other practitioners as well as the first one you see. You will find many of the answers in this book. You can go to a library or bookshop and find other books. You can get information from other patients, other hospital staff, friends, or relatives.

Much of this information will not be offered, you will have to ask and often ask more than once. If you find it hard to push for all the information, some of the following will help.

Firstly, consider taking a trusted friend or relative with you each time you see your practitioner, especially if important decisions have to be made. Two heads are always better than one. This is especially true if you are anxious and frightened. These

8

feelings are very natural and to be expected but they do make it more difficult to concentrate, think clearly and remember. The presence of a friend or relative will give you more confidence. Afterwards you will find that, between you, you have taken in and remembered much more than you would have on your own. Your friend or relative will also be in a good position to help you make decisions.

My next tip is to write down a list of questions beforehand and take them with you. Don't be embarrassed about bringing out this list in front of your practitioner—you are under stress and you have a lot to remember. Your practitioner might give you some written information but, if not, it is almost impossible to remember everything, especially if you have only been told once. Therefore, bring a pen with you and write down the information that you want to remember. If you are finding it hard to get answers that are clear enough to write down, ask again until you do. Your practitioner may try harder to be clear once he or she sees that you are determined to get the answers.

Don't feel stupid about asking for information to be explained in a different way and/or repeated as many times as you need. No reasonable person would expect you to understand and remember everything after being told only once.

Many patients hold back from asking questions because they are worried about looking ignorant or stupid. If you don't understand what your practitioner tells you it is because, whether deliberately or not, he or she hasn't explained it well enough. Communicating effectively should be an important part of your practitioner's responsibilities. He or she should be prepared to persevere until you do understand what is being said.

Nothing is so complex that it can't be made perfectly understandable by someone who is willing to share it with you. It is possible that your practitioner is so familiar with certain words that he or she has forgotten that a non-medical person doesn't know what they mean. You are not an expert and can't be expected to understand medical terms so just say if you don't understand. Sometimes a practitioner uses technical words to cover up his or her own emotions when giving bad news. You might have to help your practitioner by making it very clear that you want straight answers.

Right to as Much Time as Necessary

Are you concerned about taking up too much of the practitioner's time? He or she probably *is* busy and he or she certainly has a lot of other patients. That's the practitioner's problem, not yours. There is only one of you and it is vital that you make the right decisions about yourself. You can't do that without all the information and you need however much time that takes. If you need time by yourself or with family and friends to think things through, don't hesitate to say so and ask for another appointment. Don't be pressured into making far-reaching decisions on the spot. It is extremely rare for the situation to be so urgent that you can't take a few days to make a decision. Don't worry about inconveniencing your practitioner. You could be paying for your practitioner's services, and anyway he or she is there for your benefit, not the other way around.

Do you feel that if you ask too many questions the practitioner will label you as a 'troublemaker'? This can happen. I would say this: a practitioner who would call an anxious, responsible, questioning adult a 'troublemaker' is not the sort of person I would trust to give me unbiased information and advice, let alone make decisions on my behalf. If your practitioner is like this, then all the more reason for insisting on enough information to make decisions yourself. Alternatively, you may well think it is a very good reason to find another practitioner. I certainly would.

Right to More than One Opinion

Remember, if you find it impossible to get the information you want from your practitioner, there are alternatives. Every patient can ask for a second (or third, or more) opinion. This may be from doctors or any other type of practitioner. You may be quite happy with your practitioner's experience and technical skill but find that he or she is no good at communicating. This is sufficient reason to ask for another opinion. If the problem is with a medical specialist, you may be able to get the information through the doctor who referred you, or ask to be referred to another specialist. The referral can be from your local doctor or the first specialist. After seeing the second (or third, or more) practitioner(s) you can choose whichever one you prefer for your continuing care. You can always go back to the first one if you wish. Don't feel silly about doing this if, in the end, that is what you prefer.

This sounds easy on paper but, of course, we all know it's not. It takes courage and determination to ask for a second opinion. Many practitioners will try to talk you out of it because it is inconvenient—they may even see it as insulting. Stick to your guns. You *are* that important. You deserve the best. You're not there to protect your practitioner's ego.

If all the practitioners you see are medical doctors, they are ethically obliged to pass on all the information they have about you to the doctor of your choice. You would not need to undergo the same tests again if you changed doctors.

Don't be shy about asking for other opinions. It is very important for you to find a practitioner with whom you feel confident and comfortable. Unfortunately, in this far from ideal world, it is not always possible. If you can't find such a person, or if the treatment you want is only administered by a practitioner who is a poor communicator, you may have to use a third party to help. In this situation it would be especially important to take a medically knowledgeable friend or family member with you when you see the practitioner. Or you might have a general practitioner who communicates well with you who could serve as an 'interpreter'. He or she can get all the information from your practitioner and pass it on to you in a way you can understand.

I will stress again—*never* allow yourself to be pressured into making a decision before you understand what is involved. You can always go away, think about it, discuss it with others and then come back with your decision. It is extremely rare for a situation to be so urgent that immediate decisions are necessary.

RIGHT TO CONTROL ACCESS TO PERSONAL INFORMATION

Unfortunately, this basic and obvious right is frequently violated in the case of people with cancer. Practitioners often reveal important facts about these people to close friends or relatives without the patient's permission and, even worse, without giving the same information to the person with cancer. There can be no justification for this except where that person has completely lost his or her mental faculties. Such a person could not be reading this book, so the following applies to you.

You have the right to determine who is given information about you. Your doctor (and hopefully any other practitioner) is ethically obliged to get your permission before giving information to anyone else. It is usual to take your permission for granted in the case of other health professionals directly involved in your case. For example, other doctors, nurses, social workers, physiotherapists and so on who are personally involved in your care would not usually need formal permission to have medical and other relevant information about you. Each of these health professionals, however, is obliged to treat such information as completely confidential. The only other circumstances in which your doctor could take your permission for granted is when you bring a friend or relative into the consulting room with you. However, your doctor may think it is in your best interests not to give you all the details of your illness, while discussing your case with your close family. This is regarded as being justified, but the moment a practitioner gives information to a third person without your permission, you may feel he or she is no longer treating you as a responsible adult person.

You may know that your practitioner has already had discussions with friends or relatives in your absence. They are probably doing this in a well-meaning but misguided attempt to 'protect' you. Unfortunately the reality remains regardless of whether or not you know about it. Hiding the truth from you won't make it go away — it will just make the whole situation harder for you to grapple with.

12

I guarantee that if you are in this situation your imagination is running wild: 'It must be really terrible if they can't tell me.' I say again—your imagination will usually come up with something much worse than the truth. If you insist on being told, you are likely to get a new lease of life. You will be able to direct your energies positively into battling with a real, rather than an imaginary, situation. You will be able to share your fears and concerns freely with your loved ones. Your friends or relatives who have been given the information will feel great relief when the heavy burden is lifted from their shoulders. They also will then be able to direct their energy much more positively.

So, if you are in this situation, take your courage in both hands and make it quite clear to both your practitioner and your friend or relative that you insist on being included in all discussions like the brave, sensible adult person that you still are. Remember— secrecy divides and weakens, sharing unites and strengthens. Nothing is harder than fighting unknown terrors alone in the dark.

RIGHT TO MAKE YOUR OWN DECISIONS

While caring for people with cancer, I must have heard this phrase thousands of times: 'I suppose I'll do it if I *have* to.' I would always answer: 'You never *have* to do anything—there are always choices.'

Right to Consider Alternatives

In any given situation there is always at least one alternative. To have one treatment or another treatment or no treatment at all. To keep working or stop working, or perhaps work part-time. To stay home or go into hospital or move in with your daughter. To cry or to explode or to sulk or to smile. To talk or to remain silent. To play with the grandchildren or just watch them or stop them from visiting you at all.

Often we decide on something without consciously recognising or thinking through the alternatives. This can happen when the advantages of a particular course of action seem so great that it's not worth considering anything else. That's fine if it's true. But more often, it's best to at least go through the exercise of thinking through the possible options.

Let me give you an example. A doctor recommends a course of chemotherapy to a woman with extensive breast cancer, without offering any alternatives. For her, the alternatives in fact might include: a more or less intensive course of chemotherapy, use of different chemotherapy drugs; use of hormones; radiation treatment to the painful spots; no specific anti-cancer treatment at all; concentrating on controlling her pain with a suitable painkiller; prayer; a grape diet; or taking an overdose of her painkillers. To any one particular person, some of these will be attractive, others will be out of the question. To make the best decision, this woman needs to know the pros and cons of each alternative, and consider them in the light of her own particular life situation and beliefs. The best choice is not the same for everyone.

After getting all the information about these options, one young mother of three might decide to have intensive chemotherapy because she feels convinced that this has the best chance of prolonging her life. Another young mother of three might decide to have no chemotherapy at any stage because she has decided that, for her, the likely side effects are too great compared to the likely benefit. A third might decide to have the radiation treatment at this stage and the chemotherapy later when her symptoms come back. Each of these could be the best and most appropriate decision for each woman at that time.

As time goes by they may revise their decisions according to their own individual experiences. For example, after several months of chemotherapy, the first woman may decide the side effects she has experienced are too great to warrant continuing with it. The second woman might get to know a few other patients who have had successful chemotherapy and decide to try it herself. Again, these could be the best and most appropriate decisions for these women at that time.

Right to Decide on Your Own Treatment

Do you fully realise what I have just described? When given all
the alternatives, many people realise that the best treatment for
them is *not* the standard one recommended by their practitioner.
Why is this so? It is simply because the person with exclusive and
unique knowledge is *not* the practitioner but the patient. Never
forget this. You know much more *about yourself* than your
practitioner could ever know. You know how you feel inside: how
it feels to be in pain, or to be free of pain; to feel nauseated or to
feel ravenous; to feel listless or to feel energetic; to sleep poorly or
to sleep well; to feel black and depressed or to feel hopeful. You
know what you value in life, nobody else does.

Respect the fact that your exclusive inside knowledge makes
you, without a doubt, the best judge of what is best for you. Your
practitioner's knowledge is important, but not of this kind. It
consists of facts that can be shared. Provided these are explained
properly, there is no reason why you should not understand the
facts that are important to your case, as I have already told you.

So—find out all the alternatives, and the advantages and
disadvantages of each. Don't just let your practitioner tell you
what to do. *You* make the best decision you can at the time.
Always be prepared to revise it later in the light of new knowledge,
experience or feelings. Summed up like that it sounds easy. You
and I know it isn't: it's very, very difficult. Try anyway—remember the raft?

Difficulties in Exercising Your Right to Decide

In practice, one major difficulty is that your practitioner may not
even consider alternatives to his or her usual standard recommendation. In the last section we have discussed how you can
obtain more information. Ask for alternatives directly: 'What
would happen if I don't have what you recommend?' 'I realise you
are recommending what you believe to be the best treatment, but
what others are possible?' 'What about radiation treatment?' and
so on.

After assessing all the information yourself, you may well

.decide that what your practitioner first recommended is indeed the best choice for you. It might seem easier just to say: 'Doctor knows best—I'll do what he or she says.' Don't fall into this trap. Your practitioner has many reasons for recommending a particular treatment and I'm afraid that they do not all centre around you as a unique individual person.

Most practitioners have a series of set recommendations for various set types of patient. From their own experience and attitudes, and from the knowledge gained from their reading of the latest reports from all around the world, they decide on what they believe to be, generally, the best form of treatment for a particular type of cancer. Because practitioners are individuals with different priorities and beliefs, they do not all reach the same conclusions.

One practitioner might always think that the best treatment is the one that results in the longest average length of life, regardless of side effects. Another might prefer to stick with familiar treatments rather than to try new ones. Others try every new treatment that comes along without first critically evaluating the available evidence. Some practitioners are themselves so frightened of cancer and dying that they recommend that patients keep having intensive anti-cancer treatment even when there is no real hope of controlling the disease. Some practitioners are doing research into cancer treatment and want all their patients to have the research treatment regardless of other considerations. All that I have said in the above section applies equally to doctors and to non-medically qualified practitioners.

I know it is frightening to read all this. I know you would rather believe that your practitioner is a selfless, devoted, up-to-date saint who thinks entirely in terms of your own individual interests. Even if your practitioner were perfect, he or she could not know what issues are important to you, what your priorities and values and beliefs are. So be fair and kind to yourself. Get the information, trust your own knowledge of yourself and be prepared to make your own decisions.

Having made your decision on treatment, another major difficulty may arise. The practitioner you prefer may not be able or willing to supervise the treatment of your choice. As a general rule, it is best if your treatment is supervised by a practitioner experienced in its use. Very sophisticated treatments such as radiotherapy can be given only by certain highly-qualified medical specialists. Any practitioner is entitled to refuse to supervise a treatment that he or she believes to be useless or unacceptably toxic, or significantly worse than another treatment. Thus, the practitioner with whom you feel most comfortable may not be able to supervise your chosen treatment. You may take this factor into account in making your choice, or a compromise such as I suggested earlier may work — you may be able to get the treatment from one practitioner and the emotional support and effective communication from another, such as your local doctor.

Right to Make Other Decisions About Your Future

I have concentrated on the choice of treatment in this section as this is so important and so daunting. However, the same considerations apply to other decisions in your life as well. Naturally, you will take the opinions of other appropriate people into account. In deciding, say, whether to resign from your job, you might consider the opinions of your spouse, children, employer, fellow workers, practitioner, social worker, and priest. By all means listen to the views of people who are important to you. But, as I've said before, you are the only one who really knows what's best for *you*. Trust that.

All of the above is about the here and now. Try to apply the same ideas to the future. Have you made a will? People with cancer often avoid doing this because they somehow see it as meaning that they are giving in or giving up hope. Of course, it doesn't mean anything of the sort. All adults should have a will, because all of them, sooner or later, will most certainly die. Making a will simply means acknowledging and accepting that reality. I know that it is a reality which is unpleasantly close for you, but avoiding making a will doesn't make the possibility of death go away. If you make a will you are acting on your right to dispose of your property as *you* wish instead of leaving these

17

decisions to others who should not be responsible for them. Be strong and do it.

RIGHTS IN REGARD TO RESEARCH

Cancer research is necessary if we are to find out more about all aspects of cancer. It is quite likely that you will be asked to take part in some type of research. You need to know what your rights are in this regard.

Some research simply involves gathering facts. For example, if a researcher is trying to find the cause of the particular type of cancer that you have, you could be asked to complete a questionnaire asking about all sorts of past experiences, such as exposure to chemicals and drugs, your dietary history, previous illnesses, where you have lived and worked and so on.

Some research involves developing new tests or forms of treatment. You could be asked to undergo a new type of test which is not normally done. This would mean that they would not be sure what the results of the test mean and these results would not be of any use to your practitioner in planning your treatment. You could be asked to undergo a new form of treatment, perhaps with new drugs or a dosage or combination of drugs which is not standard. You will find more about such research in Chapter 5 of this book. At this stage, I will just detail what your rights include in any type of research.

Firstly, you are entitled to know that the procedure is experimental or unproven. You must be told the reason for the research and exactly what it would involve for you in terms of inconvenience, risk and possible side effects. You must know what the alternative standard procedures or treatments are and be assured that they are not known to be better than the research procedure or treatment. You must be assured of confidentiality —that you will not be identified by name in records going to other centres or when research results are published. You must have the opportunity to ask questions and get answers you can understand. You must be told that, whether or not you agree to take part in the research, you will still be treated by the same practitioner to the best of his or her ability. After entering the research study, you are entitled to withdraw at any stage and still receive treatment from the same practitioner if you wish. You are entitled to take time and consult with others if you wish before deciding whether or not to take part in the research. You must be assured that any adjustments or changes to treatment will be made in your own individual interest. This means, for example, that if the treatment is clearly not helping you or is producing unpleasant or dangerous side effects, it will not be continued.

Naturally, we all hope that advances will be made in cancer research. Taking part in research could be an experience which makes you feel better about yourself. You would be justified in feeling that, in this way, you could use your illness positively to help future patients. However, it is still most important to be fair to yourself and to put your own immediate interests first. Don't agree to participate in research unless you feel good about it and know exactly what you are agreeing to.

These rights are not so special or extreme, are they? They should sound familiar because, basically, they are the same sorts of rights as should apply in all treatment situations.

RIGHT TO TREATMENT BY EXPERIENCED PRACTITIONERS

Every year, medical diagnosis and treatment become more and more complicated. No one doctor can possibly know everything about the diagnosis and treatment of cancer. For this reason doctors specialise. Whenever you consider having any specialised diagnostic or treatment method you can expect to be referred to someone who is qualified and experienced in the use of that method.

For example, say you have a shadow in your lung which looks like cancer. You may be advised that, to make a diagnosis, a specimen must be taken with a needle passed through the skin and lung guided by X-rays. Make sure this is done by someone who has had plenty of experience with the method. An experienced person is more likely to succeed in getting a good specimen without puncturing your lung or causing undue pain.

You may have a cancer of the lower bowel and be advised to have this removed, leaving you with a colostomy (bowel ending in an opening on the abdominal wall). Ask to be referred to a surgeon who has done a lot of these operations. A well placed and well constructed colostomy is quite easy to look after, a poorly placed and badly constructed colostomy is a nightmare.

Say you are considering having a 'breast' reconstructed after a mastectomy (removal of the breast). Ask to be referred to a plastic surgeon who has done a lot of these operations. Only someone with plenty of experience is in a position to explain beforehand exactly what result you can expect, and then to actually produce the promised result.

All of these are just examples. If you are in doubt about the experience of your doctor, ask directly how often he or she has done the procedure in question. Ask whether there are doctors who specialise in the procedure and, if there are, ask to be referred to them.

A word of warning: specialists have advantages when it comes to knowledge, experience and technical skill. However, they also tend to have a major disadvantage—they are less likely to see you as a whole person. Specialists do not take a broad view, on the contrary, they tend to take a very narrow view. Specialists tend to see their patients as caricatures, with the particular aspect they are interested in blown up out of all proportion to everything else. They may even act as though other aspects of their patients don't exist.

Try to think of your specialists as resource people who have a lot of very specialised knowledge, some of which they can share with you. They also have special expertise which you can take advantage of, if you choose. However, even if, for example, someone knows everything there is to know about chemotherapy and is very experienced at giving it, this still does not make them the best person to decide whether *you* should have chemotherapy.

The best person to decide is someone who knows a bit about your cancer and what you can expect from chemotherapy, and a lot about you—your values, priorities, expectations, strengths and weaknesses. *That person is you.*

RIGHT TO CARE AS A WHOLE PERSON

You are a whole person with a body, a mind, a unique personality, and feelings—who happens to have cancer. I'm afraid that sometimes practitioners who treat people with cancer lose sight of this basic fact. You should expect and demand that attention be paid to all your needs. Practitioners have different reasons for working with people who have cancer. They have in common the fact that they have all chosen to battle for control over a particularly awesome and dreaded disease. They are usually involved in researching new ways of detecting, assessing and treating cancer. Many are actually very frightened of cancer and of dying themselves. Unconsciously they try to deal with their own fear by attempting to control other people's cancer and other people's lives. This means that sometimes their *own* need to control cancer and extend life prevents them from treating their patients as whole, individual people. Thus, they might press their patients to keep having intensive anti-cancer treatment when there is no real chance of controlling the cancer. They might want to feed a person with a blockage of the bowel intravenously when there is no way of correcting the blockage. They might want to keep a person in hospital having more and more tests when that person would prefer to be home. Such approaches are right and appropriate only if the person involved understands the alternatives and chooses that particular course of action. I stress again—*you* make the decision. Your practitioner can inform, recommend and advise, but *you* decide.

Another problem that can arise when practitioners become preoccupied with 'treating' the cancer is that they may not pay enough attention to your other needs. You should expect and demand attention to your symptoms, and social and emotional

21

problems. If you have pain, a cough, bowel or bladder problems, nausea or any other uncomfortable symptom, tell your practitioner. Whether or not the cancer itself can be controlled, the symptoms it produces can be treated separately. I'm not saying that you should expect your practitioner to completely rid you of all discomforts by the wave of a magic wand. I am saying that there are ways of reducing and dealing with many of these discomforts.

I know one symptom that many people do not expect to be controlled is pain. This is *not* something that everyone with cancer gets by any means, but if it does occur it *can* be treated. Don't just put up with uncontrolled pain. Ways of tackling it include radiation treatment, nerve blocks and many different painkillers. Your practitioner should be prepared to persevere in finding the right dose and type of painkiller for you. You will find more on this in Chapter 6.

Some patients don't think it 'right' to 'trouble' their practitioner with family, emotional, financial and other such problems. You have a right to help and support in these areas. Your practitioner will be interested if he or she is treating you as a person, and not just a cancer. Don't hesitate to ask. If your practitioner is not approachable and sympathetic, you may have to look elsewhere. Consider your local doctor, priest, social workers (through a hospital or social services) or community organisations and self-help groups.

This chapter is all about taking control of your life—being the ship with its captain and not the abandoned raft. I hope it's starting to sound a bit more practical! Now read on for some facts about cancer.

Chapter 2

WHAT IS CANCER?

NORMAL PROCESS OF GROWTH AND DIFFERENTIATION

Many people talk and think about cancer as if it is a single disease entity. In fact, there are over a hundred different types of cancer. They do share certain features which allow us to group them under the one word 'cancer'. However, there are many very important differences between them — they look different, start in different parts of the body, spread differently, react to different treatments, and so on.

To understand what cancer is, and why there are so many different types, we need to know something about the body's normal structure and function. We all know that our bodies are made up of many distinctly different parts. Our heart, lungs, liver, kidneys, brain, muscles, skin, etc all look quite different and all have completely different jobs to do to keep our bodies working.

Just as they all look quite different to the naked eye, so specimens from any of these looked at through the microscope can easily be distinguished from one another. Only a very small specimen is needed because the body is made up of millions and millions of very tiny units called cells. There are about 100,000 cells in a specimen 1mm across. The pathologist looking down the microscope can identify a specimen by assessing the types of cells in it and the way in which they are arranged. Cells which have different functions look completely different.

Each organ consists of a number of different types of cells arranged in a characteristic pattern. For example, the stomach has an inner lining, a muscle layer and an outer protective coat. The lining contains acid-producing and mucus-producing cells. The middle layer contains muscle cells, blood vessels with the different types of blood cells within them, lymph vessels, lymph cells, and supporting cells which hold all the others together. The outer layer contains supporting cells and nerve cells.

Some cells, such as the acid-producing cells, occur only in the stomach. Some, such as the muscle cells, are also found in the intestines, bladder and other organs. Others, such as blood and lymph vessels, are found throughout the body. Each type of cell has a unique job and a unique appearance. A muscle cell cannot do the job of a nerve cell. An acid-producing cell cannot do the job of a blood cell, and so on.

The process of developing special functions is called **differentiation** or maturation. A cell with few or no special functions is called **undifferentiated**, immature or primitive. The only function of undifferentiated cells is to multiply when necessary to produce cells which are capable of developing into specialised cells. Once cells specialise they often lose the ability to multiply. For example, mature red blood cells are so specialised for carrying oxygen around the body that they cannot reproduce themselves. As old cells wear out or are lost by bleeding, new red blood cells come from undifferentiated cells in the bone marrow, not from the mature red cells in the blood.

The normal processes of growth and differentiation are involved both in creating new human beings and in repair and renewal. Every human being develops from the union of just two specialised cells—the sperm and the egg. An embryo which is only a few days old consists of a small number of very similar looking cells. Within only a few months, these multiply, differentiate and organise themselves into a complex human being with all its different parts and functions.

Throughout life, orderly, controlled growth and differentiation continues, keeping our bodies in normal working order. The baby grows to an adult. New cells replace old, worn out ones. Injuries are repaired—after an injury cells multiply, differentiate and arrange themselves so as to reproduce the original structure as accurately as possible. For example, if you break your leg, cells which can develop into bone multiply to fill the break, mature and start to form strong bone. Damaged muscle cells, fat cells, skin cells etc are also replaced and arrange themselves so as to restore the original shape and strength of your leg as accurately as possible.

Clearly, the most incredibly complex and delicate mechanisms must exist in our body to control the normal processes of growth and differentiation. What happens if these mechanisms go haywire?

BENIGN TUMOURS

Let's start with a 'mini' form of a benign growth—warts. When the wart virus gets into cells it changes their internal structure so that they keep multiplying in an unnecessary and disorderly fashion. This forms the lump which we know as a wart. However, the wart doesn't keep on and on growing—it stops after a while. A wart is actually a very minor form of a benign growth. We use the word **benign** for growths that are not capable of causing much harm and are composed of cells which are similar to their cell of origin. If we looked at the wart cells under the microscope we would see that they looked pretty similar to normal skin cells, but they would not be quite as well differentiated. There *is* some control over the growth of these cells, they cannot damage nearby normal cells and they cannot spread to far distant parts of the body through the blood or lymph system.

There are many different types of benign growth. They can develop internally as well as on the skin—most of them can grow considerably bigger than warts! However, benign growths are usually easy to treat—in many cases it is best and easiest just to leave them alone. Removal may be recommended if they are causing cosmetic problems, discomfort or interfering with normal body functions, for example, by causing a blockage of the intestine. Also, if there is any doubt as to whether growths are benign or malignant, they should be removed or at least sampled so that they can be examined under the microscope. The cells of a benign growth are always well differentiated, that is, they look very similar to the normal cells of the organ in which they occur. Once *completely* removed, benign growths are very unlikely to grow back.

These then are benign growths. **Malignant** growths (cancer) develop when there is a much more serious disturbance of the normal relationship between our cells and the control over growth and differentiation.

CHARACTERISTICS OF MALIGNANT TUMOURS (CANCER)

Cancer growths are made up of cells which belong to our body but which have stopped behaving in a cooperative and orderly fashion. The following four features apply (with a few minor exceptions) to all malignant growths or cancers:

1. The cells cannot differentiate normally.
2. The growth of the cells is, to a large extent, outside of the body's control.
3. The cells can spread to other parts of the body (metastasize).
4. The cells can invade and damage nearby normal body cells.

Inability To Differentiate Normally

There are a great many different types of cancer. Each of the many different types of normal cells in our bodies can give rise to a cancerous growth under certain circumstances. Cancers start more often in cells which frequently replace themselves than in cells which are very stable. When we study a specimen from a cancer under the microscope we find that the cells look quite different from the normal mature cells of the organ in which the growth began. The cancer cells are bigger, and less differentiated. As you would expect from their appearance, these cells are useless. They are not capable of carrying out the special functions of the cells from which they started.

Some cancer cells are so undifferentiated that it is very difficult, if not impossible, for the pathologist to work out where in the body they originated. It is important to establish the origin of a cancer as this tells us how it is likely to behave and what treatment is likely to work against it. Therefore, the pathologist must study specimens from poorly-differentiated cancers very carefully. To establish where it started, he or she tries to find traces of the more specialised structures which occur in normal mature cells. Sometimes special techniques are used on the specimen to make such traces apparent.

There is a great deal of variation in the differentiation of cancers. Even with one cancer growth, some areas are more differentiated than others. This is one of the reasons why the pathologist might ask for another specimen if he or she has trouble making a definite diagnosis. The pathologist would be hoping to get a more differentiated specimen which contained more clues to the origin of the cells.

As a general rule, the more differentiated a cancer is, that is, the more closely its cells resemble those from which they originated, the more favourable the outlook. More differentiated cancers tend to grow more slowly, spread later and damage adjacent cells less than the undifferentiated cancers.

Uncontrolled Growth

Cancer cells have escaped the normal mechanisms by which the body controls growth and differentiation. Remember in the example of the broken leg, the cells grow and differentiate in an orderly fashion to repair the broken bone and soft tissues. Once this is done, they stop growing.

Not so with cancer cells. For a start, their multiplication has no purpose— it is not in order to replace or repair. The cells do not differentiate into useful cells. They keep growing to the detriment of the body and regardless of its normal control mechanisms. Unlike normal body cells we can think of cancer cells as uncooperative, disobedient, and independent.

Once cancer cells develop the ability to override the body's normal controls over growth and differentiation, there is another quite different natural system which may destroy them. This is the **immune system**. It consists of a complicated series of different types of white blood cells which fight together to rid the body of unwanted invaders like bacteria, viruses and so on. The cells of the immune system are also able to recognise that cancer cells are undesirable, even though they actually are part of the body and not foreign invaders. Thus the immune system has some ability to destroy cancer cells. This ability is stronger for some types of cancer than others.

One popular theory on the origin of cancer states that, throughout life, cancer cells continually develop in our body by a process of **mutation**. Mutation means a spontaneous change in the basic genetic makeup of a cell so that it is distinctly different from its parent cell. In all of us, mutations occur continually and most are harmless, but occasionally a mutation gives a cell the qualities which make it into a cancer cell—failure to differentiate, escape from growth regulation, ability to metastasize and ability to invade normal tissues. Because the change is in the cancerous cell's genetic makeup, it can pass it on to all cells which develop from it. Usually, the immune system detects new cancer cells very quickly and destroys them before they have a chance to multiply. Unfortunately, with most cancers, the immune system is only capable of dealing with a very few cells. Thus, if for some reason the cancer manages to grow to more than a few thousand cells (smaller than a pinhead), it is then beyond the control of the immune system. However, if some form of treatment destroys most of the cells, the immune system can again come in useful in getting rid of any odd ones which remain.

Many attempts have been made to artificially stimulate the body's natural immune system to deal with large numbers of cancer cells. On the whole, the results have been very disappointing.

This means that once a cancer has reached a size where it can be detected (millions of cells), it is growing independently, regardless of the body's immune system and normal controls on growth.

28

Metastasis (Ability To Spread)

This is one of the most frightening things about cancer. Cancer cells have the ability to separate from the original or primary growth, and get into blood or lymph vessels. They can then travel through the blood or lymph system to far distant parts of the body where they lodge. These cells can, in turn, multiply to form what we call secondary growths.

Understanding the Lymph System

I'll explain here what the lymph system is, because it is important in understanding cancer. When you get a sore throat you may get swollen, painful lumps in your neck. These are lymph nodes (also called lymph glands). Normally they are smaller than a pea and quite soft. There is a network of these nodes throughout your body, and they are all connected to each other by very fine channels (or vessels). Eventually, all these channels join into one which empties its contents into the bloodstream at a point just behind the inner end of your left collarbone.

The job of the lymph system is to drain all excess fluid from your tissues and to filter out any unwanted material. So, with your sore throat, the germs go through the lymph channels to the nearest lymph nodes in your neck. There they are filtered out and white blood cells get to work on them and destroy them. In the process the node gets bigger, harder and painful.

In the same way, lymph nodes will filter out and trap cancer cells which come to them through the lymph channels. The nodes actually form part of your immune system and so have cells in them which 'recognise' the cancer cells as dangerous. If only a few cells come through, they can be completely destroyed. If there are too many for the node to handle, they survive, and grow to form a hard, but usually painless, lump. This is a type of secondary growth and it, in turn, can release cancer cells to travel either through more lymph channels or the blood to other parts of the body.

29

Patterns of Secondary Growth

Your practitioner will know where your particular type of cancer usually spreads. This is very important in working out what tests are needed and what types of treatment are likely to be best. With many types of cancer, the first secondary growths to develop tend to be located in the lymph nodes closest to the primary cancer. Examples include cancer of the breast, colon and tongue. Sometimes enlargement of these nodes is noticed by the patient before there is any sign of the primary cancer.

Other types of cancers tend to release cells into the bloodstream right from the start. These include some types of lung cancer and bone cancer. For each type of cancer there is a typical pattern for locations of secondary growths. Cancers spreading through the lymph system often form secondary growths in the nodes closest to the primary. Cancers spreading through the blood often form secondary growths in the lungs, liver and bones. Although, of course, the blood goes to every part of your body, for some reason the cancer cells are much more likely to lodge and form secondary growths in some organs than in others. Thus, for example, the lungs, liver and bones are common sites while the muscles, heart and intestines are not usually affected by secondary growths.

When cancer cells lodge in lymph nodes or other parts of the body, they don't always immediately start multiplying to form an obvious secondary growth. Cancer cells have the ability to lie dormant, sometimes for many years. You could think of them as seeds which are waiting for the right conditions before they start growing. It is this ability of cancer cells to lie hidden and dormant which makes it very difficult to know whether we have completely got rid of every cancer cell. The only real test is the passage of time — we must wait until every hidden cancer cell would have started to grow and make its presence obvious. This length of time differs for different types of cancer. With some cancers we can be very confident of a cure after only two years free of any signs of disease; in others, secondary growths can still develop twenty or more years later.

Stages of Cancer

Doctors have developed a sort of shorthand method for describing how extensive a cancer seems to be. We call this the **stage** of the cancer. For most cancers there are four stages. Here are the essential things which determine the stage of a cancer. I won't go into details, but for each type there are carefully worked out rules.

Stage I cancer seems to be confined to the organ it started in. There must be no indication that it is even growing out of this organ directly into neighbouring tissues. There is only the one primary growth and, usually, this must be less than a certain size.

Stage II cancers have spread to the lymph nodes which normally drain the organ in which the cancer started. They have apparently not spread to more distant lymph nodes or through the blood. They must be confined within the nodes, not extending out of them to stick to each other or to neighbouring tissues like skin.

Stage III cancers are those which have not yet apparently spread through the blood, but *have* extended out of the organ of origin and/or the nearby lymph nodes directly into neighbouring tissues.

Stage IV cancers are those known to have already spread through the bloodstream.

The accuracy of the assessment of your stage of cancer obviously depends on how carefully you have been examined and tested. A cancer which seems to be Stage I when you have only been examined by the doctor may prove to be Stage IV after blood tests and X-rays. A cancer which seems to be only Stage II after extensive tests could still be found to actually be Stage IV when it is operated on and the surgeon can see inside. There will be more about this in later chapters.

You are probably wondering why your practitioner can't tell by a blood test whether or not your cancer has spread through the bloodstream. Remember how tiny the cancer cells are? They travel in the blood singly or in very small groups and there are only very few of them in the bloodstream at any one time. This

31

means that the chances of actually seeing them in a small sample of blood are minute. The only way we can know they *have been* in the bloodstream is by finding secondary growths in other parts of the body.

There are also some types of cancer which develop in many different places throughout the body from the start. These cancers include leukaemias, myeloma and many lymphomas. Leukaemias and myeloma begin in the bone marrow. The bone marrow is where we form new blood cells. In a child it occupies most bones but in adults it is concentrated in the central bones—spine, ribs, skull, pelvis and upper parts of arms and legs. Because leukaemias and myeloma are cancers of certain types of white blood cells, they begin where those white cells are normally formed, which is throughout the bone marrow. With leukaemias, the cancerous white blood cells can be found in a blood sample whereas in most cases of myeloma they are not released into the blood and can be found only in a bone marrow specimen.

The lymphomas are a group of cancers which originate in the lymph system. Most of these appear in many different nodes at the same time. There are some types, such as Hodgkin's disease, which tend to spread in a fairly orderly and predictable way from one group of nodes to another and, in some cases, can be successfully treated with radiation therapy directed only to the affected parts of the body.

Destruction Of Normal Tissues

Cancer cells have one other characteristic feature which is not shared by normal cells. They can invade and destroy surrounding tissues. For example, a cancer growing in a bone will replace and destroy normal bone, softening and weakening it. A cancer growing in the liver will destroy normal liver cells, reducing the liver's ability to carry out its normal job of clearing waste products from the bloodstream. A cancer growing in the lungs will damage normal lung tissues so it is harder to breathe and the transfer of oxygen into the blood is less efficient.

Normal cells exist peacefully side by side with their neighbours. Cancer cells damage and destroy them.

CAUSES OF CANCER

There is no single cause for cancer but many different factors which act together. You will remember I said earlier that it is likely that we all develop many cancer cells throughout our lifetime, but that in most cases our immune system destroys them before they have a chance to form a detectable cancer growth. The dangerous cancer cells are the ones which somehow escape the body's immune system. This escape is made possible by weaknesses in the immune system, strengths in the particular cancer cell, occurrence of a large number of cancer cells or a combination of all three.

You might understand this better if we compare it to the growth of weeds. Imagine weeds as the cancer cells and you, the gardener, as the immune system. If you check on your vegetable patch every day and pull out every tiny weed that is peeping through the soil, no troublesome big weeds will ever have the chance to form. However, if you check your garden less often or less thoroughly, or only pull out part of each weed, you'll have a problem. This is what can happen if the immune system is not working at full efficiency. Next, you could be unlucky enough to have very aggressive weeds in your garden which very quickly develop an extensive root system. In spite of careful checking and weeding every day, these particularly strong weeds might still overrun your garden. Thirdly, if a great number of new weeds appear every day, it might just be impossible to detect and pull out every one. There is no one simple reason why your garden should get overrun with weeds. It usually takes a combination of factors.

Of course, this is not to say that we can't identify some of these factors. The immune system can be weakened by other illnesses, poor nutrition, some drugs, some infections, stress, old age, cancer itself and some rare inherited disorders. Very active cancer cells can just develop by chance, but the more mutations that are occurring, the greater chance that one will lead to a cancer. The number of mutations is increased by exposure to radiation, some drugs, sunlight (skin cells only), many chemicals, and some types of infection. Exposure to any one of these factors does not necessarily lead to cancer. Thus, although we know that there are cancer-producing chemicals in cigarette smoke, not everyone who smokes gets cancer. Some smokers are lucky enough either to miss out on any mutations which lead to cancer or to have an effective immune system which prevents any cancers from developing. It usually takes more than one factor to produce cancer—unfortunately we have by no means identified them all yet.

Let me reassure you on two particular factors which worry many people with cancer.

Firstly, cancer is not inherited. You cannot pass it on to your children, even when cancer develops during pregnancy. There are a few very rare types of childhood cancer which are an exception such as retinoblastoma, a rare cancer of the back of the eye. There are also some rare inherited conditions (such as von Recklinghausen's disease, *xeroderma pigmentosa*—a rare skin disease, and some other conditions associated with multiple benign bowel polyps) which are associated with an increased risk of cancer. However, no common type of cancer is inherited. Ask your practitioner about your particular case if you are worried about this.

Secondly, as far as we know, no type of cancer is infectious. No type of cancer can be passed on directly by any form of physical contact, however intimate. However, it is true that some types of infection are linked with some particular types of cancer. For example, many, but not all, patients with a rare cancer called Burkitts' lymphoma have antibodies to one particular virus, indicating that they have been previously infected by that virus. Many, but by no means all, patients with cancer of the cervix have evidence of previous infection with a certain herpes virus. The cancer called Kaposi's sarcoma occurs in some patients with

AIDS (Acquired Immune Deficiency Syndrome)— AIDS is caused by a virus. Each of these cancers also occur in patients who have no evidence of previous infection with the particular virus involved. There is not a direct cause and effect relationship— the great majority of people who are infected with these viruses do not get cancer. As with cigarette smoking, it seems that the virus is simply a factor which can operate with other unknown factors to produce cancer in a small proportion of those infected.

TYPES OF CANCER

Cancer is classified according to the cell of origin and the organ of origin. For example, the most common type of cancer in women is called adenocarcinoma of the breast. 'Adeno' tells us that the cancer began in the cells lining the milk-producing glands in the breast. 'Carcinoma' just means cancer. There are other types of cancer which start from different cells in the breast and these have different names.

The most common type of cancer in men is called squamous carcinoma of the bronchus. 'Squamous' tells us that the cancer began in the big flat cells which line the bronchial tubes. This is the cancer we usually refer to as lung cancer but in fact there are also many different types of lung cancer, each starting in a different type of cell in the lung. The same principle goes for every other organ in the body.

It is very important to know exactly what type of cancer a person has. This is because once we know the exact type, we know how it is likely to behave— where it is likely to spread, how slowly or quickly it might develop and what treatment is likely to work against it. For example, the common type of breast cancer— adenocarcinoma— often reacts favourably to changes in the body's hormone balance. More unusual types of breast cancer, such as one starting in the fat cells of the breast, are never sensitive to hormone balance. The most common type of lung cancer— squamous carcinoma— can be cured in a fair proportion of cases by surgical removal. A slightly less common type of lung cancer—small cell anaplastic carcinoma—is very rarely cured by surgical removal, as it has a habit of spreading through the bloodstream very early.

The *only* way we can tell the exact type of cancer is by looking at a specimen under the microscope. There is more about this in the next chapter.

Wherever cancer growths are in the body, they are still named according to where the primary growth was—that is, where the cancer started. If a cancer starting in the breast spreads to the bones or liver, it is still called breast cancer, not bone or liver cancer. This is because it still looks like breast cancer under the microscope and it still acts like breast cancer. The secondary growths in the bones or liver will react to the treatments to which breast cancer reacts. A primary cancer of the bone (one starting there) would behave differently and respond to quite different sorts of treatment.

NATURAL HISTORY OF CANCER

The 'natural history' of an illness means what happens if there is no treatment. It is important to have some idea of how your cancer might behave without any treatment before you decide what, if any, treatment to have. Of course, cancer behaves in exactly the same way if it is not sensitive to the treatment chosen. Unless you are cured, your cancer will behave like this sooner or later.

As we have learnt, a cancer starts with one or a few cells. These have to double (each one split into two) about thirty times for the cancer to reach the size of a 1cm cube. It is unusual to detect a cancer smaller than this. This means that by the time a cancer is diagnosed, even when it is very tiny, it has actually been there for quite a while. It would be at least a few weeks even in the case of very rapidly-growing cancers and many months or even years for some of the slower-growing types.

Without effective treatment, the primary cancer continues to grow at a fairly steady rate, pressing on, and eventually growing through, nearby structures. Sooner or later, nearly all untreated or unsuccessfully treated cancers give rise to secondary growths. For each particular type of cancer, there is a characteristic or average pattern. For example, a cancer starting in the bone usually spreads through the bloodstream very early, and the first secondary growths are nearly always in the lungs. A cancer starting in the bowel usually takes quite a few months before it metastasizes. It then generally goes first through the lymph channels and next through the bloodstream. The first blood-borne secondary growths usually appear in the liver. Of course, as with all averages, we do not see the same pattern in every individual. One person with a bowel cancer may not have any warning signs of the disease until a complete blockage of the bowel develops. At the operation, the surgeon may find no traces of cancer elsewhere. Another person with exactly the same size primary bowel cancer could have multiple secondary growths in the liver, with no symptoms at all from the primary tumour. Everyone is different, but there are average or usual patterns to guide you and your practitioner in best planning your tests and treatment.

Just as we cannot exactly predict for any individual what organ will be affected by secondary growths, so we cannot exactly predict what will eventually cause death. Most causes of death from cancer fall into one of the two following groups. Firstly, cancer may destroy so much of a vital organ (such as the liver, brain or lungs) that it can no longer carry out its normal function. Secondly, cancer can weaken the body and immune system so much that infections such as pneumonia are fatal. These causes all act gradually. Less commonly, cancer causes death through haemorrhage, blood clots or other more sudden processes.

It is useful to think about cancer treatment as falling into two quite different groups. There are cancer treatments which can drastically change the natural course of the disease (that is, change the eventual outcome) and there are those which cannot. The first group includes all treatments which offer the possibility of a complete and permanent cure. The second group consists of treatments which temporarily arrest the cancer but hold out no chance of an eventual cure. You should insist that your practitioner tells you whether or not it is *possible* that the proposed treatment will cure you.

This is not to say that treatments from the second group are not sometimes worth having. If your cancer is temporarily arrested, this may result in you feeling better and perhaps living longer. In deciding whether or not the inconveniences and discomforts of treatment are worth the trouble, you need to know what is on the other side of the scale—the potential advantage. Many people who would put up with very unpleasant treatment if there was a chance of being cured, wouldn't consider having the same treatment for the sake of a few more months before still dying of cancer anyway.

SYMPTOMS OF CANCER

The symptoms of cancer depend on its location. I will be describing a number of possible symptoms here, none are inevitable. In Chapter 6 we will find out how to treat them. Remember that, whether or not you are having treatment to control the cancer itself, it is usually possible to do something towards relieving the symptoms it produces.

Symptoms Of The Primary Growth

Local Symptoms

First of all, what about the primary growth? Most often this is just a firm painless lump to start with. As it enlarges it may press on, or grow through, nearby structures. I'll go through some of the possible early warning signs of cancer and we'll see what causes them. Firstly, there is any unexplained **lump** or thickening that doesn't go away or is getting bigger. These lumps are usually painless. Next, any **sore** that won't heal. A cancer near the skin, or lining of the mouth, throat, bowel, bronchial tubes, bladder, womb, etc can break through these surfaces, at first just forming a raw area. If this is on the outside it looks like a sore that won't heal. If it is inside somewhere the first sign could be **abnormal bleeding** from the stomach, bowels or vagina, blood in the urine or coughing blood. Remember that blood coming from the stomach or upper bowel will come out as a very black motion, not red blood.

As the cancer enlarges it also puts pressure on, and may partly or completely block, nearby structures. If these are the bowel or bladder, a **change in bowel or bladder habit** will result. This can take the form of going either more or less often, change in consistency of the motion, an unusual amount of wind, looseness of the bowel, a feeling of needing to hurry to get to the toilet and sometimes pain on opening the bowels or passing urine. If the cancer is near the throat or bronchial tubes, pressure on these can cause **hoarseness, cough** or **difficulty in swallowing**. Pressure on the stomach can cause **indigestion**— burning, discomfort, a lot of burping, nausea or loss of appetite. Cancer starting in the skin may first be noticed as any change in a **wart** or **mole**— this includes change in size or colour, itchiness, and easy bleeding if scratched.

I can't stress too much that there are many other causes for each one of these symptoms. If you or anyone you know has one of them, it would be wise to have a checkup. If there is some other reason for them a clear report will save you a lot of unnecessary worry. If it *is* cancer, you will be giving yourself the best possible chance by picking it up early when treatment has the best chance of helping. Cancer won't go away through you ignoring the symptoms. Not doing anything about it might seem the easiest way out but this is only being very hard on yourself in the long run.

General Symptoms

As well as producing the **local** symptoms which I have described (symptoms which depend on the location of the cancer), cancer also produces some **general** symptoms. These are often vague such as lack of energy, loss of weight, loss of appetite and just not feeling your usual self. Lack of energy can be due to **anaemia** and doesn't always mean that the cancer is extensive. 'Anaemia' means not enough red blood cells to carry the oxygen around the body. You need oxygen for energy. If you have lost so much blood (and what seems like a little bit in the bowel motion every day soon adds up) that your body can't make enough red blood cells to keep up, you become anaemic. Anaemia can also develop because the presence of cancer in the body sometimes impairs the bone marrow's ability to produce blood. This can happen even when the cancer is not actually growing in the bone marrow. Another possible reason for anaemia is that some cancers make the red blood cells very fragile, so that they don't live as long as normal. Again, if the bone marrow can't keep up with the unusual demand, anaemia is the result.

There are other ways in which a primary cancer can make you feel listless and weak. Such symptoms do not *necessarily* mean the disease has spread. Some cancers release hormones or chemicals which alter the normal balance of various minerals in the blood. In this way, particular types of cancer can result in abnormally high or low levels of calcium, potassium or sodium. Such imbalances make you feel weak and are sometimes associated with other symptoms such as nausea, diarrhoea or constipation, excessive thirst and passing large amounts of urine. Successful treatment of the primary cancer will get rid of these imbalances and therefore these symptoms, provided the cancer hasn't spread. Of course, the symptoms would not be relieved by removal of the primary tumour if secondary deposits were already present.

Loss of appetite and weight can also occur when there is only a primary cancer that hasn't yet spread. This happens especially when the primary cancer is in the stomach or upper part of the abdominal cavity (liver, pancreas, spleen, etc). However, it can happen with a primary cancer anywhere.

Symptoms Of Extensive (Metastatic) Disease

Now, what about the symptoms of extensive or metastatic cancer? First of all, there are the local symptoms which depend on which parts of the body are affected. Whichever organs are involved may eventually stop working altogether.

Cancer in the Bones

If cancer affects the bones it weakens them. The weak bones break more easily than normal bones. If the spine is affected there may be pressure on the spinal cord or nerves. Such pressure can lead to pins and needles, or loss of strength in the limbs, usually the legs or feet. Cancer in the bones is not always painful. Sometimes one or two spots are painful while others which look very similar on an X-ray are not. Even if the cancer itself can not be controlled there are a number of different ways of dealing with the pain (see Chapter 6).

Cancer in the Liver

If there are secondary growths in the liver, they will gradually replace it. Until over ninety per cent of the liver is destroyed, it is still possible for the remaining cells to do its normal job. The liver's job is complicated but basically consists of purifying the blood by clearing out various waste products, drugs, etc. The liver also makes some substances which help the blood to clot normally. If less than ten per cent of the liver is functioning, the patient gets yellow jaundice — the eyes and skin look yellow because bile-like substances are not being cleared properly from the blood. (Yellow jaundice also develops when there is a blockage of the bile system, for example, with gall stones — it does not necessarily mean a disease of the liver itself.) Because the blood does not clot as well as normal, a patient with a failing liver bruises and bleeds easily. Fluid tends to accumulate in the body, especially in the abdominal cavity. Often there is no pain because pain only occurs if the cancer deposits break through or stretch the sensitive outer lining of the liver. As the liver enlarges it tends to press on the stomach, causing loss of appetite and sometimes nausea. There are drugs which can help this. Gradually impurities build up so much in the blood, that the patient becomes tired and drowsy and eventually loses consciousness altogether and dies.

Cancer in the Brain

If cancer involves the brain, the first signs may just be symptoms of raised pressure within the skull—headache, vomiting and maybe blurred vision. Of course, there are many other possible reasons for these symptoms. Contrary to what many people imagine, cancer in the brain very rarely causes the complete alteration in personality which some people call 'madness'. Its effects depend on which part of the brain is involved. For example, if a cancer growth is in the part of the brain that controls the left side of the body, the patient can lose the ability to use the left arm and leg normally. This usually develops gradually and may be accompanied by numbness and/or twitchy movements of those limbs. Some patients have convulsions just like those that epileptics have. These can usually be prevented with the same drugs as we use for epileptics. There is treatment which can reduce the pressure on the brain, and in some types of cancer treatment can temporarily shrink the growths. Once cancer has spread to the brain however, it can never be permanently cured. Eventually the growths produce such a high pressure on the brain that the patient gradually loses consciousness and dies.

Cancer in the Lung

Cancer in the lungs causes difficulty in breathing. The job of the lungs is to put oxygen into the blood and take waste gases such as carbon dioxide out. If part of the lung is destroyed, the rest of the lung has to work harder to do this. This means the patient needs to breath faster and gets puffed out easily on exertion. Breathing extra oxygen, especially at times of exertion, helps the lungs to get enough oxygen into the blood. Other symptoms may include a cough and wheezing. As with the liver, pain is not common. It only occurs if the cancer grows through or stretches the sensitive outer lining of the lung. This lining is called the pleura (it is what gets inflamed in pleurisy). Sometimes, breathlessness is due to fluid forming outside the lung. If this happens it is often possible to take the fluid off with a needle or tube through the skin. This can give very good but temporary relief as the fluid will form again unless the cancer that is producing it can be successfully treated. Breathing extra oxygen allows the damaged lung to get enough oxygen into the blood only up to a certain point. If too much of the lungs are destroyed, oxygen in the blood drops and carbon dioxide builds up, gradually causing drowsiness and loss of consciousness and death.

Some General Effects of Extensive Cancer

Extensive cancer causes some general effects throughout the body, in addition to the symptoms due to involvement of particular organs. Weight loss is due to a combination of loss of appetite, and the fact that the cancer cells use up a lot of the available nutrients. However, many people die of cancer without ever losing much weight at all. Like pain, weight loss is by no means something that occurs in every case.

Cancer also tends to weaken and suppress the body's immune system. This means that infections are easily caught and tend to be more serious than they are in a person without cancer. Because of this, infection, which often takes the form of pneumonia, is a frequent cause of death in cancer patients.

There are also ways in which cancer can cause sudden death. One is through bleeding, which is often internal. Another is through blood clots on the lung. Blood clots form more easily in people with cancer than in people without cancer. Blood clots can travel to the lungs and lodge there. This can completely block the blood flow through the lungs, in which case death occurs within minutes. If the clots are not big enough to block the blood flow completely, the symptoms consist of shortness of breath, chest pain and coughing of blood.

With cancer we have seen that death is often due to failure of the liver, brain or lungs to do their normal job. In the case of the lungs this may be due to cancer itself, pneumonia or blood clots. In all these instances, it is unusual for the patient to remain fully alert and conscious up until the time of death. In fact, it is most unusual for patients with cancer to suddenly drop dead, whatever the actual cause of death. A gradual drifting into sleep and un-

43

consciousness, usually comes first. In most cases, especially if everyone is prepared for it, this is best for both patients and their loved ones.

If you've read right through this chapter to here, you're a very brave person. Stick with it! Now that we know something about what cancer is and how it behaves, let's find out what to do about it.

Chapter 3

DIAGNOSIS OF CANCER

DIAGNOSIS IN PEOPLE WITH SYMPTOMS

It is possible to find some types of cancer before any symptoms have developed, that is, while a person is still perfectly healthy and has noticed absolutely nothing wrong. This is discussed at the end of this chapter. However, most cases of cancer are diagnosed after one or more symptoms have developed. I described many of these early warning symptoms in the last chapter.

How do we go about finding the cause for such symptoms? There are two essential, basic steps. First, we have to find some way of actually seeing the source of the problem. Second, if it looks at all suspicious of cancer, we have to obtain a specimen to be examined under the microscope. A word that is often used in referring to the trouble spot is **lesion**. This is a general word which covers any abnormality, not just cancer. Because it is so general it is a useful word to use when we don't know exactly what the problem is.

ACCESSIBLE CANCERS

The cancers that are easiest to diagnose are obviously the ones on the outside. Thus, if there is a sore that won't heal on the skin, in the mouth or anywhere else where it can easily be seen, it's just a matter of the doctor looking at it. If it looks at all suspicious of cancer a specimen is taken. This may sometimes be done by gently scraping some cells from the surface. However, such a specimen may only contain a mixture of blood cells, germs and dead cells which cannot be identified. This means that it is often necessary to get a specimen from deeper down. This can be done with a needle or by actually removing a small piece of the lesion under a local anaesthetic.

Some cancers start very close to the surface and can be seen and felt as a lump under the skin by the patient and the doctor. Common ones are cancers of the breast, lymph nodes (primary or secondary), and testicle. A lump under the skin can be the first indication of other cancers also, such as ones starting in fatty tissues, muscle, bone etc. Of course, there are many other possible causes besides cancer for lumps under the skin.

If you show your doctor such a lump, he or she will firstly want to know the history of it. If it has only been there a short time (weeks to months) and is getting bigger this would be more suggestive of cancer than if it had been there for years and was staying the same size. Most cancer lumps are *not* painful. Next your doctor should carefully examine the lump for its size, hardness, tenderness and exact location, checking whether it is attached to any organs. At this stage, your doctor may be able to tell you quite definitely that it is not cancer. If there is any suspicion, it is necessary to take a specimen, either with a needle through the skin, or by actually removing all or part of the lump under a local or general anaesthetic.

There are some places that you can't see but your doctor can see quite easily. There are simple instruments to help your doctor look quite painlessly up your nose, down your throat as far as the voice box (larynx), into a woman's vagina as far as the neck of the womb (cervix) and 20cm or so up your back passage (anus and rectum). So, for symptoms like a blood-stained discharge from the nose, cough, hoarse voice, coughing blood, irregular vaginal bleeding or bright blood in the motions, your doctor can check the appropriate part in the surgery at your first visit without any anaesthetic. In some cases, he or she may also be able to take a specimen then and there. For example, in the case of vaginal bleeding, a smear test can be taken and may provide a definite diagnosis when examined under the microscope. If there is a lump or ulcer in the anus or rectum, a tiny specimen can be taken with forceps in the surgery quite safely and painlessly.

INTERNAL CANCERS

Visualising The Cancer

Often, however, your doctor will not be able to give you the answer so quickly. For any problem that is more internal than those I have mentioned so far, more complicated methods are needed to get to see the source of the symptom.

Endoscopic Methods

There are instruments available now that allow us to see parts of the body that we previously could only see by operating or (indirectly) by X-rays. These instruments are basically long flexible tubes that can be passed into various passages. They have a sophisticated lighting system that can 'see around corners' and often also magnify any abnormalities that need closer checking. The specialist can also take specimens through them. This means of looking inside is called endoscopy ('endo' means inside, 'scopy' means looking at). In 'upper gastrointestinal endoscopy' we go through the mouth and see into the throat, gullet (oesophagus), stomach and upper part of the small intestine, and even, in some cases, into the tubes from the liver, gall-bladder and pancreas. With bronchoscopy, also done through the mouth, we can see down the windpipe (trachea) into all the major bronchial tubes of the lung. With colonoscopy we go through the anus to see the whole of the large intestine (colon). Cystoscopy is going through the urinary passage (urethra) to see the bladder and opening of the tubes from the kidneys. Most of these examinations are usually carried out with the patient awake. They are uncomfortable but shouldn't be painful. Your doctor will usually give you a sedative to help you relax. Of course, any of these can be done under a general anaesthetic but this is not quite as safe.

Similar instruments have been developed for looking into some of the body cavities. This is nowhere near as major a procedure as an actual operation. The laparoscope (or peritoneoscope) can be inserted through a small cut in the abdominal wall. Through this the doctor can see the outside of many organs such as the liver, spleen, intestines, urinary bladder, ovaries and uterus (womb). A similar instrument called a thoracoscope can be used to look at the outside of the lungs. With mediastinoscopy, an instrument is inserted through the skin of the neck to look down behind the breastbone at some of the lymph nodes which drain the lung.

The main advantage of endoscopic methods is that they are safe. They may be uncomfortable but they do not involve radiation, surgery or (usually) general anaesthetics. The main disadvantage is that they require sophisticated, expensive equipment and experienced people to operate them. This means that they are not always available. Like all methods they are also not foolproof— abnormalities may be missed, even by experienced operators. Endoscopic methods are not available for every part of the body. One way and another, it is often necessary to use other methods instead of, or as well as, endoscopy.

Simple X-rays

X-rays are one means of looking indirectly at internal organs. Just what are X-rays? They are a form of electromagnetic radiation. Other electromagnetic rays include ordinary light, infra red, ultraviolet, radio and TV waves. These are all forms of energy which can travel through space in straight lines but differ in wavelength and frequency.

Light is the one that is most familiar to us, simply because light is the only one that the human eye can detect. To help you understand how an X-ray picture is produced, we can use an example involving a form of electromagnetic radiation that we all understand—light. Imagine a light shining through a stained glass window onto a white wall. On that wall you can see a 'picture' of the window. The picture is formed because light gets through some parts of the window more easily than others. No light gets through the frame or the lead separating the pieces of coloured glass. Some light gets through the glass but the amount depends on the strength of the light and the thickness and colour of the glass. The detail we get in our indirect 'picture' depends on these factors. Exactly the same sort of process is involved in getting an X-ray picture. The X-ray machine sends out X-rays like a source of light. The X-rays get through some parts of our body more easily than others. Because we can't see X-rays with our eyes, instead of a white wall on the other side we need an X-ray plate. The X-rays react with the special coating on the X-ray plate to form a 'picture' which we can see. X-rays travel most easily through air and least easily through very solid things like metal and bone. Just as we can use a stronger light to get more detail, so we can adjust the machine to send out 'stronger' X-rays if we need more detail.

So, for example, what do we see on a chest X-ray? The air in the lungs and around the body looks black, because all the X-rays get through the air. The heart and big blood vessels look greyish-white (a few X-rays get through). The bones of the ribs and spine look very white (hardly any of the X-rays get through). A solid area in the lung is easy to see. It looks white against the black of the air in the normal lung around it. Weaknesses in bones are also fairly easy to see—more X-rays get through the softer bone. The weakened part shows as a grey area in the normal white bone. Because very few X-rays get through bones and some of the larger organs, it is often necessary to take X-rays from more than one angle to get a complete picture. For example, if we want to 'see' the part of the lungs that lies behind the heart we need to take an extra X-ray from the side of the body as well as the front-to-back one.

Unfortunately, in many parts of the body it is very hard to see an abnormality on a simple X-ray. This is the case when the abnormality lets through as many X-rays as the normal part, because it is the same density. For example, cancer spots in the kidney are not much harder or softer than the normal kidney. On an X-ray they come out white and so does the normal kidney.

This means you can't see them. The same applies to the brain, liver, stomach, bowel, pancreas and many other organs. What can we do to overcome this problem?

X-rays using Contrast Methods

The internal structure of many organs can be made to show up on X-rays by using contrast materials. These are usually substances which are much denser than the normal tissue (that is, let far fewer X-rays through). Barium is such a substance. If you swallow a liquid barium mixture, it coats and fills the gullet and stomach. Later on, the small intestine will be lined by the barium as it passes through. Any ulcers or growths then show up as dark irregularities against the white of the barium lining these organs. If something is pushing on, say, the stomach from the outside, this will also be seen — the white barium inside the stomach shows whether its shape and position are normal. Fizzy substances can also be swallowed to produce contrast. In this case the contrast is provided by a less dense substance — air. The air looks black and when used in combination with barium provides a 'double contrast'. A similar mixture can be put into the rectum by enema to outline the large intestine (colon).

Other contrast methods involve the injection of very dense liquids (often iodine-based) into the bloodstream. X-rays taken immediately after injection show up the blood vessels themselves as white lines (this is called angiography). We can see whether the blood vessels are partly or completely blocked or displaced from their normal position. Sometimes we can show up extra blood vessels which could be feeding a cancer growth.

In addition to showing blood vessels, we can also use injected contrast materials to show the internal structure of organs like the kidney and gall-bladder system. For the kidneys, we inject a substance which can be passed out of the body through the urine. Soon after injection the internal structure of the kidney will be outlined with dense white as the kidney extracts the contrast material from the blood. A little later X-rays will show the tubes going from the kidneys to the bladder and then the bladder itself, as the contrast material passes through in the urine. Abnormalities in these organs may then be seen—for example, a kidney stone might show as a dark patch in the white contrast material. A cancer growth in part of the kidney could distort or partly block the drainage system. If the kidney had stopped working altogether, no contrast would appear in it at all. There is some sort of contrast method available to help us see the details of nearly every organ in the body.

Computer Assisted Tomography (CT Scanning)

In recent years computers have been linked up to very sophisticated X-ray machines to produce a more detailed and quite different type of picture than those I have described above. The pictures which this system produces look like a cross-section of the part of the body under study. This means that they represent what you would see if you sliced the body right through at a particular level and looked at the cut surface. The usual type of X-ray is produced by a broad beam of X-rays passing through the entire part of the body to be checked. With the CT scanner, a very narrow beam of X-rays passes backwards and forwards across the body in a thin strip. Instead of an X-ray plate on the other side there are special crystals which react very quickly to X-rays falling on them. Messages are constantly being fed into a computer telling it how many X-rays went in one side (from the X-ray source) and how many came out the other side (as indicated by the reaction of the crystals). By analysing these messages sent from every angle around the body, the computer builds up the cross-sectional picture. The process can be repeated at other levels in the body as necessary. CT scan pictures give us much more detail than an ordinary X-ray. Contrast methods are often used in combination with the CT scanner to give the maximum possible information. The problem with CT scanners is that they are extremely expensive and need expert staff to 'read' the pictures. They also involve the use of considerably more radiation than normal X-rays.

Radiation is of course a problem with all forms of X-rays. The rays are not completely harmless. *Unlike* light and the other forms of electromagnetic radiation, X-rays are a form of ionising radiation.

This word 'ionising' means that the X-rays are capable of damaging the actual molecules of substances that they pass through. The amount of damage depends on the 'strength' of the X-rays and the length of exposure. There is no amount of radiation that can be guaranteed as absolutely safe but it is believed that the amount of radiation involved in taking X-rays has only a very minute chance of causing problems such as cancer in the future. Every effort is made to keep the radiation to a minimum. Much research has gone into developing equipment that will take good X-rays with the least possible amount of radiation going through the patient. The rays only pass through you for a very short time while the machine is turned on. Your doctor and X-ray specialists between them should ensure that X-rays are taken in such a way that they get the maximum information for the least possible amount of radiation. Ask them about this if you are worried. They should tell you why the X-rays are being taken, what information they will give, and why it is important to have this information.

Radio-isotope Scans (Nuclear Medicine)

This is a completely different way of using ionising radiation to get pictures of internal organs. Instead of sending X-rays through the body from an X-ray machine *outside* it, these pictures are produced by rays coming from tiny amounts of radioactive substances *inside* the body. Although this probably sounds less safe than X-rays, the amount of radiation involved is often less than with X-rays of the same part of the body.

Say, for example, we want to get a picture of the liver. One of the liver's normal jobs is to keep the blood pure by removing certain substances from it. When such a substance is injected into the blood, it is concentrated in the liver within a short time. If that substance has been made radioactive, it sends out rays through the body which can be detected with something similar to an X-ray plate. The picture produced in this way shows us the shape, size and location of the liver and which parts are working normally. Any part of the liver which has been so badly damaged that it can't do its normal job will show up as a 'hole', where there is little or none of the radioactive substance.

The substance used for bone scans is taken out of the blood by bone-forming cells, and concentrates especially in areas where the bone cells are very active. In this type of scan, abnormalities show up not as 'holes' but as 'hot spots'—areas where *more* than the usual amount of radioactive substance collects. This is because bone cells are especially active around abnormalities such as fractures, infections, or cancer deposits. The scan picks up the problem indirectly by showing the bone cell reaction rather than the abnormality itself. The amount of radiation involved in taking a scan of all the bones in the body is actually quite a bit less than if all those bones were X-rayed.

Various radio-isotopic methods can be used to get 'pictures' of most organs. For different organs we use different substances, choosing one that will be concentrated in the particular organ we wish to study. In all cases the radioactivity does not stay in the body for long. It is passed out through the urine, faeces or air from our lungs. The amount of radioactivity involved in each test is very small, and doesn't pose any danger to anyone you go near or touch. If you want exact details, ask the people who are doing the test. They should tell you how long it takes your body to get rid of the particular substance being used and which way it is eliminated.

One drawback with these tests is that you only 'see' the parts of the organ that are functioning normally. The 'holes' or 'hot spots' can be due to any one of many things that interfere with that organ's function. Cancer is only one of many possible reasons for abnormalities in these scans.

Methods for Indirectly Visualising Internal Organs Not Involving Radiation

I'm sure you've heard of the depth-finders that ships use. These instruments send out a beam of ultrasound waves. By measuring how long these waves take to bounce back from the ocean floor, the depth at that point can be worked out. Ultrasound waves are *not* electromagnetic. They are the same as sound waves but of a frequency and wavelength that the human ear cannot pick up. They bounce back off some surfaces just as sound waves bounce back as echoes from cliffs.

Ultrasound can be used in medical diagnosis, because it bounces off some tissues in the body more readily than others and passes through different body tissues at different speeds. A machine that produces ultrasound waves is placed on the skin overlying the part of the body to be checked. The 'picture' formed by the waves echoing back can be 'read' by experienced people, but is not as clear as those of X-rays and scans. This method was developed originally for pregnant women because of the great importance of avoiding radiation to the delicate foetus. It is now used for many other purposes. Because it doesn't involve any radiation it is especially useful when repeated examinations are needed, for example, to check the effects of treatment on a growth. However, it can only be used on certain parts of the body and only shows up certain types of abnormalities clearly. Ask your doctor if you want to know more about its possible use in your particular case—it may or may not be suitable and/or available.

Thermography is a means of getting a 'picture' of various parts of the body by measuring the amount of heat coming off. For example, a thermographic picture of the breast might show excessive heat coming from a known lump. This would mean the lump was unlikely to be a fluid-filled cyst and more likely to be cancer or an abscess. This method is not very reliable because many factors can influence the amount of heat coming off different parts of the body.

Surgery—Emergency and Planned

In some cases, cancer is diagnosed during surgery. Sometimes the first indication of a cancer is an emergency necessitating an operation. Previous warning symptoms may have been ignored or incorrectly interpreted. In some cases there simply are not any earlier warning symptoms. The emergency could take the form of blockage of the bowel, heavy bleeding into, or from, a growth or perforation (the cancer breaking through the wall of, say, the bowel, allowing the contents to leak out and cause peritonitis). At the operation, the surgeon will do what he or she can to correct the emergency situation, take samples of the cancer for microscopic examination and check for signs of any secondary spread. At least it means we get a direct look at the cancer when this happens!

Occasionally, when there is very strong suspicion of cancer but no tests give definite proof, it is recommended that the patient have an exploratory operation. If this is suggested to you, remember that planned operations are safer on the whole than emergency ones. However, don't agree until you are satisfied that this is the best step to take. Alternatives might include repeating inconclusive tests at a later date or making further attempts to get a sample of suspicious areas without going to the lengths of having an operation.

Getting A Specimen

We now know most of the ways of getting a direct or indirect look at the source of symptoms which might be due to cancer. Once the problem area is located, the next step is to obtain a sample for microscopic examination. *This is always necessary.* Even if the appearance on X-rays, say, is such that your doctor is perfectly sure it's a cancer, it is still necessary to *confirm* this *and* to find out what *type* it is. Until this is done, no one can know what to expect, how to best treat it or anything else. I cannot stress this too strongly—it is always necessary to examine a specimen under the microscope. What are some of the ways of getting the specimen?

Exfoliative Cytology

'Exfoliative' means falling off (like leaves off a tree). 'Cytology' means the study of cells. When a cancer breaks through any surface, cells fall off it singly or in little clusters. For example, a lung cancer which has grown through the lining of a bronchial tube sheds cells which may be coughed up. Examination of sputum (spit) specimens under the microscope may reveal cancer cells. Cells from cancer of the bladder can float off and be found in specimens of urine. Cells from cancer of the uterus (womb) or cervix (neck of the womb) may be found in samples taken from the surface of the vagina and cervix (a Pap smear). When the diagnosis is made by this method, we can sometimes be in the position of knowing that a cancer is present before we have 'seen' it by some other means. For example, a sputum specimen from a patient who has been coughing blood sometimes shows cancer cells when the X-ray looks quite normal (that is, the cancer is too small to show up on the X-ray).

Exfoliative cytology is a quick and easy way of making a diagnosis when it is positive, that is, cancer cells are found. However, when it is negative, that is, no cancer cells are found, it is not so helpful because cancer may still be the cause of the symptom. Some cancers don't release cells at all, or only release them now and then, so clear specimens do not necessarily mean no cancer. Other tests would be necessary to make a definite diagnosis.

Aspiration Cytology/Needle Biopsy

'Aspiration' means sucking up. Cytology, as you know, means the study of cells. We all know what needles are! Biopsy literally just means getting a specimen from a live person. The above terms are used to describe getting a specimen from a suspicious area with a needle. With aspiration cytology, a very fine needle is used and the specimen consists of separate or very small groups of cells. With a needle biopsy, a special type of slightly larger needle is used and a tiny solid sliver of tissue is obtained. If the lesion is just under the skin, the needle goes through the skin. Sometimes needle specimens are also taken through the vagina or rectum. Local anaesthetic (numbs the area but doesn't put you to sleep) is used and the procedure should be no more painful than a blood test. If the specimen is to be taken from an area that is not an easily felt lump, the test may be carried out under X-ray control, to make sure the right spot is sampled. This applies, for example, in needle biopsies of the lung or some bones.

Aspiration cytology and needle biopsy specimens must be

taken with special types of syringes and needles by persons experienced in this method. Even then, because only a few cells from one small part of the abnormal area are in each specimen, the diagnosis can be missed and repeat specimens may be necessary. As with exfoliative cytology, a clear specimen doesn't rule out cancer.

This method can obviously be used only when the suspicious area is in a place that is easy and safe to get at.

One special type of needle biopsy is the bone marrow test. The bone marrow is a soft red jelly-like area in the centre of many bones. This is where new blood cells are formed. Bone marrow cells can usually be sucked out quite easily using a fine needle. If the narrow cavity is scarred or packed with cancer cells, it may not be possible to get a liquid specimen. In these cases a tiny solid sliver of bone and marrow can be taken with a special, slightly larger biopsy needle. The pelvic bone can be used for both types of specimen. The breast bone, being easier to get at, is often used when only a liquid specimen is needed. Again, provided plenty of local anaesthetic is used to numb the sensitive outer covering of the bone this procedure should not be very painful.

Most bone marrow conditions are generalised, that is, they occur throughout the bone marrow. This means it doesn't usually matter which particular bone the specimen comes from.

Incision and Excision Biopsies

'Incision' means cutting out part of, 'excision' means cutting out the whole of an abnormal area. This can be done with scalpels etc in the form of a mini-operation or with special forceps and other instruments designed to neatly nip off a tiny sample. Such instruments are available for taking specimens from internal lesions through endoscopy tubes. Because of this, endoscopy is a very useful type of test—we can see the abnormality and get a specimen from it in the one procedure. In many cases, these specimens are from spots which, in the past, could only have been biopsied at a full scale operation. Endoscopy can be uncomfortable, but it's certainly much safer, simpler, more convenient and less painful than an operation!

As I explained in the previous section, if lesions can't be reached through the skin or by endoscopy, an operation may be necessary to get a specimen. As with every type of specimen that consists of only a small fragment of the abnormal area, incision biopsies are only helpful if they are positive, that is, give a definite diagnosis. A negative biopsy can only rule out cancer when the whole lesion is removed and examined under the microscope. An excision biopsy may be recommended whenever a conclusive diagnosis cannot be made using the other methods I have described. In the case of enlarged *lymph nodes*, it is usually best to remove one completely anyway. This is because lymph node conditions can be diagnosed much more accurately and reliably when the pathologist can see the pattern of the whole node and not just a few cells from one part of it.

Blood Tests

You may have been wondering why I have made no reference to **blood tests** yet. This is because blood tests are rarely useful in making a definite diagnosis of cancer. You remember the two essential steps in diagnosing cancer don't you?— 'seeing' the source of the symptom and taking a specimen. Blood tests are no use for either of these unless the cancer actually starts in one of the types of blood or lymph cells. With leukaemias, some myelomas and some lymphomas, enough malignant cells travel in the bloodstream to allow a diagnosis to be made by looking at a small sample of blood under the microscope. Even so, specimens from bone marrow or lymph nodes are usually necessary as well.

You may well ask: 'But don't many types of cancer spread through the bloodstream?' Indeed they do. The problem is that only a few cells at a time are released from the primary cancer and they don't stay in the blood for long. The chances of actually seeing them in a small blood specimen are minute. It can happen but it's very rare.

Blood tests sometimes help by giving us clues as to where to look when cancer is suspected.

Of course, they are also very important in assessing how extensive and serious the situation is once cancer is definitely diagnosed. Blood tests are necessary to check the function of all the organs, the strength and purity of the blood, the balance of different minerals and hormones in it and so on. There is more about all this in the next chapter.

There are practitioners who will tell you they can definitely diagnose cancer, or even the tendency to cancer, on a blood test. With the following exceptions, *this is not true*. Firstly, as I have explained, the actual malignant cells can be seen in the blood in leukaemia, and sometimes myeloma or lymphoma. Secondly, there is a particular rare type of cancer of the testes (malignant teratoma) which can release a hormone into the blood called *h*uman *c*horionic *g*onadotrophin (HCG for short). This hormone is normally found only in the blood of pregnant women. When found in a man's blood it definitely means that man has this particular type of cancer. I know of no other instances where cancer can *conclusively* be diagnosed by a blood test. There are other cancers which can release large amounts of certain chemicals and hormones into the blood. When these chemicals and hormones are discovered by blood tests they do make your doctor very suspicious of cancer. However, with the one exception of HCG in a male, there are always other possible causes for these abnormalities. They can only be put down to cancer after the cancer is located and biopsied.

Some practitioners also claim to be able to diagnose cancer by testing your hair. *This is not true*. Like finger and toe nails, hair consists mainly of a substance called keratin. There are no cells in hair—it is not living tissue. It is not possible to diagnose cancer by analysing hair.

DIAGNOSIS IN PEOPLE WITHOUT SYMPTOMS—SCREENING

If you've read everything up to here, you will know why there is no simple screening method for cancer. Unfortunately, we can't just line everyone up once a year and do a simple test which picks out all the ones with early cancer. Even when cancer is well established, you now know that the diagnosis can involve a lot of complicated, time-consuming, inconvenient and expensive tests. If only there *was* a simple blood test — how easy things would be!

Screening means looking for a condition in normal healthy people who have no symptoms. An ideal screening test would have the following features:

1. Simple, safe, cheap and convenient.
2. No false negatives, that is, would not miss any cases.
3. No false positives, that is, would not pick up conditions other than cancer in mistake.
4. Capable of picking up the condition at a stage when it is completely curable.

Screening for Lung Cancer

Let's see how close we could get to this for, say, lung cancer. Screening tests we could consider are sputum cytology, X-rays and bronchoscopy. Sputum cytology is simple, safe and convenient for the patient. However, each specimen takes quite a few minutes to examine thoroughly and this must be done by a specially trained technician, so it is not cheap. There are false negatives — not all cancers shed cells into the sputum to be coughed up. Some do so erratically — there may be no cancer cells in the specimen that goes to the laboratory even if there were the day before and the day after. False positives are rare but occasionally other abnormal cells are mistaken for cancer cells. The test *can* pick up very tiny cancers at a stage when surgical removal would have a good chance of curing the patient. To pick up very early cancers, specimens would have to be examined every few months, which obviously would make it extremely expensive in the long run. Another problem occurs if the cancer is so small that it can't be seen on X-ray. It then has to be located by bronchoscopy or special types of X-ray before it is possible to go ahead with surgical removal.

How about X-rays for screening then? These are not completely safe, especially if we consider repeating them every three or four months for years on end. They are simple and convenient but not cheap. False negatives can occur if the cancer is small or situated close to the heart and major blood vessels, making it hard to see. False positives are more common than with cytology, as a number of other conditions can produce similar shadows. Additional tests would be needed to confirm the diagnosis. The smallest cancer we could hope to see would be about a centimetre across, often they would be bigger. The chance of completely curing these cancers by surgical removal is not so good, as some will already have spread.

Bronchoscopy is so expensive, inconvenient and uncomfortable that it couldn't really be considered as a screening test for large numbers of patients. Remember that it would have to be repeated every few months if we wanted to get all the cancers early. Cancers in the small bronchial tubes or in large ones but not ulcerating through the lining would be missed—those false negatives again. False positives are rare. This test can pick up cancers at a stage where they are surgically curable, but some would already have spread.

Although this all sounds so discouraging, lung cancer screening programmes have been tried. A high-risk population was chosen for testing—males over forty-five who were heavy smokers. X-rays and sputum cytology were repeated every four months. Some early cases were picked up and operated on successfully, but there were still patients who developed symptoms of cancer between screens, that is, in the four month breaks. Some of the cases picked up at screening had already spread. The numbers of patients eventually dying of lung cancer were not convincingly less than those for a group of men who were not screened regularly. Therefore, for lung cancer at least, there is so far no effective method of screening.

Let me stress that all of the above refers to patients with *no symptoms*. All I am saying is that patients diagnosed by these screening methods did no better in the long run than patients who were diagnosed and treated *as soon as* they developed symptoms. The screening tests weren't good enough. They only picked up the same proportion of curable cancers as are picked up in patients who go to the doctor *as soon as* they develop symptoms. Don't take this to mean that you shouldn't go and have tests if you have any symptoms that could be due to cancer. The longer you leave it, the worse your chances. With many types of cancer, the only cases that are ever cured are the ones that haven't spread before diagnosis and treatment. The later cancer is diagnosed, the more likely it is to have spread.

Screening for Cervical Cancer

There is one type of cancer where screening almost certainly does make a difference to the outcome and that is cancer of the cervix (neck of the womb). Why is this so when it isn't for our previous example of lung cancer? One reason is that most of the cervix can be easily seen with a speculum (internal examination). Cells can be gently scraped from the outer part of the cervix and from the part that we can't see on internal examination—the small inner canal leading to the womb. This is the Pap smear which, when correctly taken, contains samples from all parts of the cervix to be examined under the microscope. What we cough up does not contain cells from every part of our lungs. The cells in the lung samples are only those that have fallen off by themselves, with the Pap smear they are gently scraped off. Next, the cells of the cervix go through a recognisable pre-cancer stage. This means that cells which are very likely to develop into cancer if left untreated can be identified under the microscope in the Pap smear. It takes quite a few years for pre-cancer to develop into actual cancer which can spread. There is a pre-cancer stage for lung cancer too but it is probably shorter and the cells are not often seen in cytology specimens. The next thing is that effective treatment is more possible if pre-cancer or cancer cells are found: part of or all of the cervix can be removed. We can remove part of the lungs but we can't remove them all, for obvious reasons. Thus with cervix cancer it is fairly easy to get comprehensive samples for cytology tests, it has a longer and more readily identified pre-cancer stage and it can be effectively dealt with once diagnosed (by complete surgical removal). These are the factors which result in screening picking up a higher proportion of curable cases than happens if we wait until patients get symptoms.

While mentioning Pap smears, I'll just take the opportunity to tell you that a clear Pap smear (when properly taken) only really rules out cancer of the cervix. Cancers of the uterus (womb) and ovaries are rarely diagnosed on Pap smears—it is a screening test only for cancer of the cervix.

A lot of research has gone into screening for breast cancer. There is some evidence that yearly screening with clinical examination (feeling the breast) and mammography (special X-rays) in women over forty-five may improve the survival for breast cancer, but it doesn't make a dramatic difference. I believe the best way of ensuring that breast cancer is diagnosed as early as possible is by examining your own breasts regularly and reporting to a doctor when you detect any lump or thickening. Breast cancer diagnosis is often delayed because women who *know* they have a lump 'keep an eye on it' themselves for some time before seeking attention. What I say about this applies to every symptom that may be due to cancer. If it is *not* cancer, having tests right away will put your mind at rest and save you a lot of unnecessary worry (most breast lumps are *not* cancer). If it *is* cancer, the earlier it is diagnosed, the better your chances. Pretending it isn't there won't make it go away—it will only give it more time to grow and spread.

Cancer of the cervix is the only type of cancer where a screening procedure has been shown to influence the mortality of the disease. You could think through possible screening procedures for other types of cancer yourself—I think that the examples I have given are enough to show you the difficulties involved. If only there was a simple blood test for cancer!

Chapter 4

ASSESSING THE EXTENT
OF THE CANCER

Making the diagnosis of cancer is only the first step towards establishing the outlook and the best way of caring for a person with cancer. To do this, we usually need to know exactly which parts of the body are affected by cancer and how severely. Depending on what treatments are being considered, it may or may not be advisable to track down every last cancer deposit.

Basically, tests to determine the extent of a cancer should be done only if the results would influence your treatment and care. Keep this in mind when tests are being arranged. Ask your doctor to explain the reasons for the tests he or she recommends, especially if you can't see what difference their results would make. Some doctors keep arranging more and more tests rather than face up to telling a person that their cancer cannot be cured, or some other unpleasant news. They do this to protect themselves, and at your expense. Don't let them get away with it. Only agree to tests that are being done for a good reason that *you* understand.

It is not always important to know the exact extent of the cancer. The importance depends on what treatment is being considered. For example, say a woman and her doctor were considering an extensive operation to remove the entire womb and both ovaries for cancer of the cervix. It would be important to be as sure as possible that there were no traces of cancer in other parts of the body before doing such an operation. A number of tests would be advisable to check thoroughly for possible secondary deposits.

What if this woman was found to have secondary cancer deposits in her bones? After finding out about the possible alternatives, she could decide to have no actual anti-cancer treatment and to concentrate simply on relief of symptoms. In this case, whether or not she also had cancer deposits in the lungs or liver would make no difference to her treatment, unless she had symptoms which could be originating in these organs. It would also be unnecessary to know exactly which bones were affected, as long as they were not causing pain. Tests to determine the exact extent of her cancer would be unnecessary.

On the other hand, she might decide to have chemotherapy treatment. In this case, tests to find out how well her liver was functioning might be necessary in order to work out the right dose of chemotherapy drugs. It wouldn't be necessary to know just how many secondary deposits there were or which particular bones or other organs they were in, because the chemotherapy drugs would travel right through the body anyway.

There are three separate aspects to think about when assessing the extent of cancer—we need to know the extent of the primary growth, of lymphatic spread, and of blood-borne spread.

EXTENT OF PRIMARY GROWTH

If surgical removal or radiotherapy treatment aimed at completely eradicating the cancer is being considered, it is very important to check the extent of the primary cancer very carefully. In all other situations it is not usually important to know the exact extent of the primary growth.

Surgery and radiotherapy are both local forms of treatment. This means that they act only where they are applied and not in other parts of the body. Obviously they have a chance of being successful only if all of the cancer is within the treated area. A lung cancer starting near the heart and extending into it would not be cured by removing the lung. Radiotherapy for the same lung cancer would have no chance of controlling it unless the heart was included in the area being treated. Local treatment cannot be properly planned until the local extent of disease is known. To assess this, the doctor must first find out exactly what symptoms the patient is having and then examine him or her carefully. Depending where in the body the primary growth is, endoscopic methods, X-rays, scans or other tests might also be useful. For example, if a patient with lung cancer complains of chest pain, the doctor should suspect that the cancer has grown out of the lung into nearby structures because cancer in the lung itself is not painful. With or without pain, bronchoscopy, mediastinoscopy, ordinary X-rays and CT scanning are tests which should be considered before deciding to go ahead with surgery. Surgical removal of part or all of the lung should not be attempted until it is fairly sure that removal of the whole cancer is possible.

The same sorts of considerations apply to cancer in any part of the body. By taking a history of symptoms, doing a careful clinical examination and arranging appropriate tests your doctor should have an accurate idea of the extent of the primary cancer *before* surgery or radiotherapy is commenced. Even so, the surgeon may still discover only after opening the patient up that complete removal of the cancer is not possible. This can happen even after the most careful pre-operative assessment. Of course, the chances of it happening are greatest when the pre-operative assessment is least thorough.

Remember that the extent of the primary growth is only important when local treatment is planned. As a rule, if secondary growths are known to be present and/or if treatment which goes right through the body is to be used, it is not necessary to know the exact extent of the primary growth.

ASSESSMENT OF LYMPHATIC INVOLVEMENT

You remember the lymph node system that I described in Chapter 2? How can we check whether or not the cancer has spread through this system?

Normal lymph channels are like cotton threads. Normal lymph nodes (glands) are soft, smaller than a pea and cannot be felt through the skin. If cancer gets into the lymphatic system it usually grows in the lymph nodes, making them bigger and harder. This is usually painless.

Much less often, lymph spread takes a different form—the cancer can actually grow in the lymph channels. If the affected channels are in the skin, the appearance is usually that of a raised, red 'rash'. One of the most troublesome sites for this type of spread is in the lungs. The solid cores of cancer cells running through the lymphatic vessels make the lungs very stiff. This causes coughing and shortness of breath. Unfortunately this problem can be hard to diagnose, because it is often difficult to see on an X-ray in the early stages.

If the cancer fills the nodes or blocks the lymph channels, it prevents that part of the lymph system from carrying out its usual job. One of these is to drain excess fluid from the tissues. So, for example, if the affected nodes are in the armpit, the arm may swell up.

Evidence of Lymphatic Spread

The first way to look for evidence of lymphatic spread is simply to carefully examine the patient, checking for swelling of the tissues and enlarged nodes. Because the lymph network nearly always follows the same pattern, your doctor will know which particular group of lymph nodes to check most thoroughly. For example, if the primary cancer is in the arm, or breast, the first lymph nodes to be affected would be those in the armpit. From there the cancer can go into the lymph nodes in the part of the neck just above the collarbone on the same side. There are lymph nodes just under the skin in the neck, arm pits, crease of the elbow, groins and back of the knee. If any of these are enlarged, they can easily be felt.

Unfortunately, there are many lymph nodes that are not so conveniently located. Chains of lymph nodes run up from the groins, just in front of the spine through the abdomen and chest. There are also groups of lymph nodes near most of the internal organs. Channels from these lead into the main chain I have described. They eventually form one large channel which empties its contents into the blood vessel just behind the inner end of the collarbone on the left. Cancer in a node at this spot can come from almost anywhere in the abdominal cavity or chest. Lymph nodes do not show up on normal X-rays. The only exception is some in the chest which, when enlarged, can be seen against the black air in the lungs. However, there are several ways of getting 'pictures' of the other internal glands. CT scanning is one method. This works best in chubbier people in whom the lymph nodes tend to be surrounded by fat. Because fat lets through more X-rays than the lymph nodes, it provides a contrast which allows us to 'see' the nodes more easily than in a thin person. In thin people the nodes lie next to muscles and blood vessels, both of which let through about the same amount of X-rays as the nodes themselves, making them very hard to 'see'.

Lymphangiography

Lymphangiography is another means of showing up lymph nodes. For this a liquid form of contrast is injected into the tiny lymph channels and gradually works its way up through them. For example, if the 'dye' is injected into lymph channels in the foot, within a few hours X-rays will show it in the channels as far up as the groin and abdominal cavity. The next day the nodes themselves will be filled with the contrast material, sometimes right up into the chest. Their size and internal structure can then be checked. Unfortunately, because lymph nodes which are packed with cancer don't function normally, the contrast may not get into the worst affected nodes. This can be a major drawback of this test. It is less likely to happen with lymphomas than with other types of cancer. Combining both methods by doing a CT scan *after* injecting the contrast actually gives the maximum information.

The biggest drawback of lymphangiography is that it can be used to show up only certain groups of nodes. Unless the nodes we want to 'see' are fed by channels which are accessible (to have the contrast injected into them) we cannot show them up by this method.

Thus, lymphangiography cannot be used to show the lymph

nodes from many of the internal organs such as the bowel, bladder, womb etc. Often it is only during an operation that we can easily find out for sure whether or not these are affected.

Lymphomas

Cancers actually *starting* in lymph nodes are grouped together under the name lymphoma. In turn, lymphomas are subdivided into two groups — Hodgkin's disease and non-Hodgkin's lymphomas. Each of these groups contains a number of quite different subtypes. Hodgkin's disease tends to start in one group of nodes and spreads in a fairly orderly and predictable way to other groups. Most non-Hodgkin's lymphomas tend to develop in many different groups of nodes at the same time, although there are a few particular types which spread like Hodgkin's disease. All lymphomas can also affect the bone marrow, liver, spleen and other organs.

Lymphomas can be treated by radiotherapy or chemotherapy. Hodgkin's disease and a few particular types of non-Hodgkin's lymphoma can be completely cured by radiotherapy, provided *every* involved node is treated. Here it is extremely important to track down every single deposit of the disease. In contrast, if chemotherapy is to be used, it is not as important to know where the disease is, because the chemotherapy drugs go right around the body anyway.

ASSESSMENT OF SPREAD THROUGH BLOODSTREAM

It would be wonderful if we could tell by a simple blood test whether or not cancer cells have got into the bloodstream. You will remember from Chapter 2 that it is very rare to actually see cancer cells in a blood sample. There are never many of them in the blood at any one time except in leukaemia and some cases of lymphoma and myeloma. The chances of seeing cancer cells in the tiny drop of blood that is looked at under the microscope is minute. Because it is so hard to 'catch them in the act', the usual way of finding out that cancer cells have *been* in the blood is by finding the resulting secondary deposits.

Most of the tests that we use are only capable of picking up cancer deposits that are more than about 1cm across. You might remember from Chapter 2 that cancer cells can go through the blood, lodge somewhere in the body and lie dormant there for a long time. These tiny dormant seedlings are made up of only a few cells and cannot be detected by currently available tests. We only find out later that these cells have been there—when they activate and grow into a deposit that can be detected. If your doctor tells you that your tests are clear and no secondary growths have been found, this is certainly good news. However, it is not a cast-iron guarantee that there will be no trouble in the future. The danger period during which dormant seedlings can activate is different for different types of cancer, ranging from as little as twelve months to as much as twenty or more years. Ask your doctor how long it is for your particular type of cancer.

You may well ask: 'If they can't see cancer cells in the blood, why on earth do they do so many blood tests?' Blood is a very complicated mixture and there are many different tests that can be done on it. It can be looked at under the microscope to check the proportions, numbers and appearance of the different types of blood cells. The number of red cells and their ability to carry oxygen can be measured. There are many tests to determine whether the blood can clot normally. A large number of different hormones, minerals, proteins and waste products can be measured, enabling us to check the function of many organs in the body. They don't do every possible test on each sample of blood, but only the tests your doctor asks for. Abnormalities will only be found if the right test is requested.

How then does your doctor decide what tests to recommend when looking for possible blood-borne secondary deposits? Firstly, he or she searches for clues by checking your symptoms, and examining you carefully. Secondly, your doctor should know how your particular type of cancer usually spreads. Thirdly, he or she should consider whether or not the result of each proposed test would make a difference to your care. The doctor must combine knowledge about your type of cancer in general with knowledge about you in particular in order to best decide what tests to recommend.

These three considerations should be in your doctor's mind continually from when he or she first sees you. They apply at every stage of the disease, but especially at decision-making points. These points include, of course, when the cancer is first found but also whenever a change in treatment is being considered. The change could be to start, stop, or change treatment directed against the cancer itself, or to alter symptomatic treatment (treatment directed at relieving symptoms, without attacking the cancer).

The most common sites for blood-borne secondary deposits are lungs, bones, liver and brain. Some types of cancer are more likely to go to one of these sites and some have other 'favourite' sites. Ask your doctor what the usual pattern is with your particular type of cancer.

Lung Metastases

Symptoms which might make your doctor suspect lung secondaries are breathlessness, coughing (especially coughing up blood) and chest pain. Your doctor may well want to check your lungs even if you have none of these symptoms. This is because they are such a common site and because secondary deposits here may be quite big before they produce any symptoms. Also it is easy to check the lungs—firstly by clinical examination, and secondly with a chest X-ray. Your doctor examines the lungs firstly by tapping his or her fingers. The lungs should sound hollow because they should be full of air. If part of the lung is solid or filled with fluid, it won't sound hollow. Next, your doctor listens with the stethoscope, to check the sound of your breathing. If the bronchial tubes are narrowed, a whistling sound may be heard through the stethoscope. If part of the lung is not working, the sounds of air moving in and out will be absent there. If the lining of the lung is roughened, a rubbing sound may be heard. Your doctor may ask you to say something—usually 'ninety-nine'—while he or she listens through the stethoscope. This is because the sound of your voice travels better through solid lung than through fluid.

While this examination can give useful clues, a clear examination does not always mean that the lungs are normal. For example, if a number of small secondary deposits are scattered throughout the lungs, most of the lung is actually working quite normally. There may be no symptoms nor abnormalities on clinical examination. A chest X-ray is always necessary when looking for lung secondaries.

You'll remember that the air in the lungs makes it quite easy to see any abnormalities. The secondaries can take the form of fluid outside the lung or solid deposits in the lung. With fluid on the lung, the cancer cells are not actually in the lung itself but in the outer covering. This covering is called the pleura—you will have heard of pleurisy which is the name for inflammation of this covering. If cancer cells (or germs or other types of inflammation) damage it, the pleura reacts by producing fluid which lies outside the lung itself. On an X-ray the fluid forms a white patch right across the side of the chest that it is on. In severe cases it can even make one whole side of the chest look white. This happens if the fluid takes up so much space that there is no room for air in the lung. Both to relieve symptoms and to confirm that it is due to cancer, your doctor might recommend removal of some of the fluid. This is usually easily done through the chest wall using a needle or rubber tube. If it is due to cancer, microscopic examination of the fluid will usually show cancer cells.

When secondary cancer in the lung is in the form of solid deposits, an X-ray usually shows them as round white shadows against the black air of the lung. If it is especially important to know whether or not there are lung secondaries, a CT scan may be recommended to look for spots that are too small to show on a plain chest X-ray. Often the appearance is so typical that there is no need to go any further to prove what they are. However, if they don't have the typical appearance or they are unexpected for your type of cancer, your doctor may recommend that you have an aspiration biopsy. A fine needle can be inserted into one of the lesions through the skin, under X-ray control. The diagnosis can then be definitely proved if cancer cells are found in the specimen. Of course, as I mentioned in Chapter 3, if no cancer cells are seen, this does not prove it is *not* cancer.

If you have a lung biopsy, there is a small risk that air will keep leaking out of the lung afterwards. Some air always leaks into the pleural cavity, but usually the hole seals over quickly. There is also a small risk of internal bleeding. Your breathing, pulse rate and blood pressure should be checked regularly after a lung biopsy. An X-ray may also be recommended the following day to check that the leak has sealed. Small amounts of air that get into the pleural cavity are not a problem. The air gradually gets absorbed back into the system. However, if a lot of air leaks out of the lung, the lung collapses and doesn't function properly. If this happens, a plastic tube may have to be put through the chest wall into the pleural cavity to drain the air out until the leak seals over. This may take some days. The risk of this should be discussed with you before you have a lung biopsy. It is more of a risk if you have emphysema. Ask the doctor about the risks if he or she doesn't tell you.

Bone Metastases

What about the bones—how do we check for secondary deposits there? Pain is the most common symptom that leads your doctor to suspect cancer in the bones. However, the pain may just be in one bone when a number are affected and sometimes there is no pain at all. In some cases the diagnosis is made only after a fracture in a weakened bone occurs. However, it is very rare for a fracture to occur at a site that hasn't been at all painful beforehand.

If the cancer in the bones fills up a lot of the bone marrow cavity, this prevents you from making new blood cells normally. Any one or all three of the red cells, white cells and platelets may be affected. Too few red cells is anaemia, which can make you tired and lacking in energy. Too few white cells makes you liable to get infections more easily than normal. Too few platelets means the blood doesn't clot properly, so that you bruise and bleed easily.

Blood tests can be done to check the numbers of these cells. The fact that the anaemia, low white cell or platelet count is due to cancer in the bone marrow may be suspected when the blood is examined under the microscope. The bone marrow is full of immature forms of each of the blood cells. When this cavity is filled with cancer cells, the immature bone marrow cells can be 'pushed out' into the blood before they have differentiated into mature blood cells. If these immature cells were seen in your blood, your doctor would be very suspicious of cancer in the bone marrow. However, other cells in the marrow cavity can also cause this—the most common is scar tissue. Immature cells may also be released into the blood when there are unusually heavy demands for new blood cells. This can happen after bleeding, with severe infections, and when the blood count is recovering after having been reduced by chemotherapy or other drugs. If your doctor thinks cancer is the likely cause, a bone marrow examination might be recommended to make sure.

Besides the blood count, other blood tests can help your doctor when looking for evidence of bone secondaries. Large amounts of a certain enzyme called alkaline phosphatase may be released into the blood by active bone cells. (An enzyme is a special type of protein which keeps cells functioning normally by helping certain types of chemical reactions.) The enzyme alkaline phosphatase helps bone cells produce new bone. It also helps other cells in the body to function normally, especially liver cells. When the cells are either very active or damaged, some of the enzymes they contain can leak into the blood. Cancer in the bones is only one of the possible reasons for high alkaline phosphatase levels being found in the blood. Other causes include fractures, infections in bone and all sorts of liver problems. A high alkaline phosphatase doesn't prove anything in itself, but is a clue that should lead to other tests to find the reason.

Cancer in the bones can also cause the release of large amounts of calcium into the blood. This can cause nausea, vomiting, loss of appetite, metallic taste in the mouth, constipation, muscle weakness, excessive thirst and the passing of large volumes of urine.

Again, there are a number of other possible causes for high blood calcium levels which your doctor would have to consider.

If bone secondaries are suspected, X-rays or bone scans, or both, may be necessary. X-rays of a bone secondary may show a weakened area which looks darker than the normal white bone, because there is less calcium in the affected spot. Sometimes, however, the nearby normal bone reacts very strongly to the presence of cancer cells, producing a calcium-rich area that looks whiter than the normal bone. After successful treatment, healing bone secondaries can also look like this. In some cases bone secondaries do not show up on normal X-rays at all. Quite a lot of bone has to be destroyed before they can be seen. A CT scan of the suspected area is more sensitive, and may be positive when the plain X-ray looks normal.

Bone scans are a very useful means of looking for secondaries. They can also pick up cancer deposits in bones which look normal on plain X-ray. A spot which has hardly weakened the bone at all still produces a reaction in the normal bone cells nearby. It is in these active bone cells that the radioactive substance is concentrated. Thus the bone scan can detect cancer deposits which are at an earlier stage than those visible on a plain X-ray. The problem is that the bone scan shows up all reactive bone cells regardless of the reason for the reaction. Fractures (recent or old), arthritis and infections also can show up on bone scans as 'hot spots'. Bones which show 'hot spots' on scan usually have to be X-rayed to find out what is causing them. Occasionally the normal bone cells do not react to cancer cells nearby. In this case the bone scan will be falsely negative, that is, will miss the cancer spots. This happens especially with myeloma. The most reliable way of looking for bone secondaries is with a combination of bone scan and X-rays.

Liver Metastases

The liver is often the first organ affected by metastatic deposits when the primary cancer is in the stomach, intestines, pancreas or gall bladder. Many other cancers can also spread to the liver. Symptoms can include nausea, loss of appetite, bloated feeling in the upper abdomen, jaundice, itchy skin, and passing dark urine. Of course, there are many other possible causes for each of these symptoms.

The liver is situated just under the rib cage on the right. When it is enlarged, it can be felt. Because it moves down when you take a deep breath, your doctor may ask you to breathe deeply while he or she is feeling for the liver. Tapping over the liver also helps to determine its size. The liver is solid and therefore gives out a dull note when tapped. Because there is air in the lung above it, and usually some air in the intestines below it, these areas sound hollow when tapped. The size of the liver is estimated from the extent of the area that sounds dull.

When the liver is damaged, fluid tends to collect in the abdominal cavity. This is called ascites. One reason is that cancer or scarring in the liver can partly block the blood and lymph vessels. In addition, the liver normally produces a blood protein called albumin. If the liver doesn't keep the albumin in the blood up to normal levels, fluid leaks out of the blood into the tissues. This can cause swelling in the legs or lower back as well as fluid in the abdominal cavity. Ascites in a person with cancer does not always mean the liver has secondary deposits in it. Cancer cells growing in the lining of the abdominal cavity (the peritoneum) also causes fluid to collect, just like the fluid on the lung when the pleura is affected. Of course, problems other than cancer can cause ascites too.

When checking for clues to the presence of cancer in the liver, your doctor would also be looking for yellow jaundice, which is seen most easily in the whites of the eyes.

Whether or not liver secondaries are suspected, on the basis of symptoms and clinical examination, blood tests to check the liver's function may still be recommended. This is because even a normal sized liver in a person who feels quite well may still contain small secondary deposits. The enzyme we mentioned before when talking about the bones—alkaline phosphatase—is one that would be checked. There are also other liver enzymes that can be measured. In addition, certain waste products are checked. These are the yellow substances that cause jaundice when they build up in the blood. Slight build ups that are not enough to be seen as jaundice can be picked up on blood tests. Slight reductions in the amount of albumin in the blood do not cause fluid problems. Thus, even if there is no swelling or ascites, it is worth checking the albumin level. Particularly if a liver biopsy may be needed, certain tests to check whether your blood is clotting normally may also be advised. This is because the liver produces some of the proteins which help the blood to clot.

Tests that allow us to 'see' the liver are not necessary in every person with cancer. They are usually only recommended when there are clues from symptoms, clinical examinations or blood tests that there is liver abnormality. A radionuclide liver scan shows us the size of the liver and whether there are any areas in it that are not functioning normally. Normal X-rays do not show up the liver. A CT scan does and it may also pick up cancer deposits as they let through less X-rays than the normal liver. In some cases, the combination of symptoms, clinical findings, blood tests and scans build up a picture so typical of liver secondaries that a biopsy for conclusive proof may not be recommended. However, when there is something unusual or unexpected about the situation, or when it is very important to be quite certain, a liver biopsy should be considered.

This can be done with a special type of needle through the skin, under local anaesthetic. Because the liver moves up and down as you breathe, it is important to try hard to hold your breath when the doctor asks you to. Before doing a liver biopsy, your doctor should make quite sure that your blood can clot normally. If not, injections can be given to correct this. Even so, it is possible to bleed internally after a liver biopsy. This is unusual, but has to be watched for carefully. After the biopsy you will be kept lying still for some hours while the tiny hole in the liver seals over. During this time your pulse rate and blood pressure should be checked regularly. The main danger of bleeding is right after the biopsy. Sometimes transfusion is necessary. Very rarely, an operation is needed to stop the bleeding.

Central Nervous System Metastases

The central nervous system is the brain and spinal cord. Blood-borne metastases to the central nervous system most often take the form of solid round lumps in the brain. Cancer cells can also lodge and grow in the covering of the brain and spinal cord. This covering is called the meninges (you have probably heard of meningitis, which is inflammation of this covering). This covering encloses the cerebro-spinal fluid (CSF), which surrounds and cushions the entire brain and spinal cord.

Cancer in the central nervous system produces symptoms by two completely different means. Firstly, the cancer growths interfere with the function of the part of the brain or spinal cord that they are growing in or near. Secondly, as the cancer deposits grow, they cause a build up of pressure in the whole central nervous system. This happens because the brain and spinal cord are completely enclosed in solid bone—the skull and vertebral column. As the cancer grows, pressure builds up because there is hardly any room for things to enlarge.

What happens when cancer growths interfere with the function of the brain or spinal cord? Most often there is simply loss of function of whichever part of the body is controlled by the affected area. Thus, if the cancer growth is in the left side of the brain, there may be loss of feeling and strength in the right side of the body. A growth in the spine pressing on the spinal cord can cause paraplegia—loss of feeling and strength in the legs and loss of control of the bladder or bowel. As well as loss of function, cancer growing in the brain can irritate the brain cells, causing twitching or convulsions. This does not happen with lesions in the spinal cord or meninges.

The symptoms of increased pressure in the brain and spinal column can include headache, nausea, vomiting, blurred or double vision and stiffness in the neck and back.

Your doctor should examine you carefully for any loss of feeling or strength, especially if you have any of these symptoms. He or she should also examine the back of your eye, by looking through your pupil with a special lighted instrument called an ophthalmoscope. The end of the optic nerve can easily be seen at the back of the eye with the ophthalmoscope. The optic nerve is actually an out-pouching of the brain itself. Build up in pressure on the brain can cause the end of the optic nerve to swell, producing a typical appearance, which your doctor should recognise. Unfortunately, however, the optic nerve *can* look quite normal even when the brain pressure is very high, so this is not a foolproof test.

As a rule, tests to check the central nervous system are only recommended if there is good reason to suspect a problem there. One exception is in certain types of leukaemia and lymphoma, which have a high chance of spreading to the meninges. With these, it is advisable to check for meningeal involvement right from the start. If the tests are clear, preventative treatment may be recommended as part of a treatment plan aimed at curing the cancer altogether.

Normal X-rays do not show up the brain or spinal cord at all, because they are completely enclosed in bone. A radio-isotope scan is one way of 'seeing' the brain. Unlike for liver and bone, the substance that is injected is not concentrated in the brain cells. What it actually shows up are the areas that have more than the usual amount of blood flowing through them. Cancer deposits show up because they nearly always have a greater blood flow than the normal parts of the brain. The CT scan is another way of showing cancer deposits in the central nervous system. The deposits usually let through less X-rays than the normal brain and spinal cord.

These X-rays and scans show up cancer lumps but do not help much when looking for meningeal involvement. To check for this a lumbar puncture is necessary. Under local anaesthetic, a fine needle is inserted into the fluid which surrounds and cushions the spinal cord and brain (the cerebro-spinal fluid or CSF). The pressure in the CSF can be measured through the needle and is an indication of the pressure throughout the central nervous system. A sample of fluid can be withdrawn for testing, including examination under the microscope for cancer cells. When done correctly, a lumbar puncture is not much more painful than a blood test. Headache can occur after a lumbar puncture. These headaches are thought to be due to CSF continuing to leak out through the tiny hole in the meningeal covering. To reduce the chance of this happening, you may be advised to lie flat for some hours after the lumbar puncture.

Central nervous system symptoms can also result from cancer deposits pressing on a part of the central nervous system from the outside. Thus, a deposit starting in the bones of the spine or between the bone and meningeal covering can cause pressure on the spinal cord. Because the outside part of the meninges is called the dura, these deposits are called extradural lesions ('extra' meaning outside of). Symptoms depend on the location. They often include pins and needles, loss of feeling and loss of strength in the feet and legs, and partial or complete loss of control of bowel and bladder. Extradural lesions cannot be seen on a plain X-ray. They do show up on a CT scan. Another way of 'seeing' them is with a myelogram. Here a liquid contrast material is injected into the spinal fluid through a lumbar puncture needle. Because the liquid is heavier than the spinal fluid, it 'settles' in the lowest available location. The person can be safely tilted up and down at different angles on a special 'tilt table' to get the contrast material to the trouble spot.

I have discussed in detail how we can look for secondary deposits in the common sites: the lungs, liver, bone and central nervous system. The same type of approach applies to whatever part of the body is suspected of containing secondary lesions. Suspicions based on symptoms, findings on clinical examination or blood tests may be followed up by appropriate X-rays, scans, biopsies etc. Ask your doctor for an explanation if you don't understand why certain tests are recommended. You have every right to refuse tests, for example, if you can't see what difference the results would make to your care.

UNKNOWN PRIMARY

So far in this chapter we have considered the approach when we start from the primary cancer. What happens when we have to deal with the reverse situation? It is not unusual for the first indication of the presence of cancer to be in the form of secondary growths. For example, the chest X-ray of a person who complains of coughing blood may show a number of small secondary cancer deposits. A person who has slipped over and broken the thigh bone may be found to have a secondary cancer spot at the site of the fracture. Nausea, loss of weight and upper abdominal discomfort may lead to the diagnosis of secondary cancer in the liver. In such cases we have to work backwards taking clues from the secondary deposits to help in our search for the primary cancer.

The same basic considerations apply here—tests should only be considered if the result would make a difference to the person's care. We must consider whether knowing where the primary cancer is will make any difference to treatment. Local forms of treatment aimed at eradicating the cancer are clearly out when there are already secondary growths. Forms of treatment which go right through the body (chemotherapy, hormone therapy, etc) may be useful for certain particular types of cancer, so it is worth searching for these types (see later chapters). If symptomatic treatment only is being considered, there is no point in searching for a primary cancer that is not causing any symptoms. We can wait for the symptoms and deal with them if and when they develop.

You will remember from the last chapter that the crucial step in diagnosis of cancer is to get a sample of the suspicious area for examination under the microscope. This is also true for people with probable secondary deposits and unknown primary. Examination of such a sample is usually necessary to confirm the diagnosis of cancer. In addition, by studying the shape, size, type and arrangement of cells from the secondary growth, the pathologist can often suggest likely primary sites. In deciding what further tests to recommend your doctor should consider the appearance and location of the secondary deposits, common cancer types for your age and sex and what treatments might be possible as well as the pathologist's advice. Once you have ruled out primary cancers which are sensitive to certain particular hormone, chemotherapy or other treatments which go right through the body, there is rarely anything to be gained by searching further for the primary tumour. It may reveal itself later by producing symptoms which can then be dealt with. However, in some cases the primary cancer never causes any problems and is not located before death results from the effects of the secondary growths.

Well, that wasn't such a difficult or unpleasant chapter, was it? You now have enough background to start thinking about treatment. First of all, it is important for you to understand *why* certain treatments are recommended. It is also important to understand what sorts of things you will need to know in order to decide whether what is recommended is likely to be best for you. This is what the next chapter is about. It is an extremely important chapter. *Don't miss it.*

Chapter 5

CHOOSING YOUR TREATMENT

INTRODUCTION

If you've read this far, you are obviously keen to understand your disease. You are prepared to face the reality of being an adult person with a serious illness. You don't want to be treated like a helpless young child. You deserve and expect explanations.

That's great, as far as it goes. But I hope very much that you are not content to stop at that. I hope that you take it one step further, and use this understanding and knowledge as a stepping stone that enables you to make your own decisions. I can well imagine you are doubtful about taking this further step. Perhaps you're thinking: 'It's nice to understand what's happening, but surely it's easier and safer to leave the decisions to the experts?'

I know that's what you've been taught to believe. I know that's what you want to believe. But I also know that enormous numbers of cancer patients have suffered because they have believed it. I know that a great many cancer patients undergo unpleasant and pointless tests and treatments because they unquestioningly accept the decisions of experts—both medical doctors and other practitioners. I also know that it is extremely difficult for patients who *do* want to make their own decisions to get the necessary information. These are my reasons for writing this book. I don't want *you* to suffer in this way. I hope that by the end of this book you will understand why the decisions of experts are often not the best decisions for people with cancer. I hope you will believe that *you* are the best person to make decisions about yourself. I hope you will have enough confidence and understanding to ask the right questions and get the information you need to make the best decisions for you.

Believe me, I wish there was an easier way for you. However, let's carry on and see how we can deal with this reality you're stuck with.

In this chapter I will be explaining how your doctor decides what treatment to recommend, why this may not actually be the best treatment for you, what difficulties to expect in getting the information you need and how to make sense of this information once you've got it. This chapter explains *why* I think you need to decide for yourself and how you can go about doing this.

In the next chapter I will discuss symptomatic treatments. These are treatments aimed not at curing or controlling the cancer, but at controlling the symptoms of the cancer. Here we will look at how problems such as pain, lack of appetite, nausea, coughing, constipation and so on can be tackled.

In the following four chapters I will give you more details about the types of treatment which I believe are capable of controlling or curing certain types of cancer. These are surgery, radiation therapy, chemotherapy and hormone therapy.

I will not be discussing in detail at any stage other cancer treatments such as laetrile, cleansing and alkalinising diets, heat treatment, faith healing, prayer, meditation, developing a positive mental attitude, herbal remedies and so on. This is partly because I have no personal experience with using these forms of treatment. In addition, I don't believe they have a high chance of controlling or curing any type of cancer or that they are the best way to control the symptoms of cancer. That is *my* own belief—*you* must come to your own conclusions. Although I am giving you details only of the treatments with which I have personal experience, I hope I am also giving you the basic information, vocabulary and concepts which will help you to explore any type of treatment you wish.

WHY THERE IS NO MIRACLE CURE FOR CANCER

I have explained that there is no simple reliable test for cancer. In the same way, I'm afraid there is also no single, simple, reliable treatment for cancer—no treatment which we can rely on to eradicate every cancer cell in every patient. In your heart of hearts I'm sure you know that's true—otherwise why are so many different treatments promoted? The fact that there are such a bewildering number of treatments recommended simply means that no one of them is a wonderful, highly effective and reliable cure for every type of cancer. This is not to say that there are *no* effective cancer treatments. There *are* treatments which have a very good chance of curing or controlling *particular types* of cancer, but there is no single treatment which works against every type of cancer.

Why is this so? Firstly, as you now know, there are many different types of cancer. As well as differing in appearance, where in the body they start, when and how they usually spread and so on, they also differ in how they react to treatment.

Thus, surgery has a good chance of curing some types of cancer, but only those which are usually still confined to the primary site at the time of diagnosis. Cancers which tend to release cells into the bloodstream or lymphatic system before they are diagnosed are unlikely to be cured by surgery. Other types of cancer are extremely sensitive to radiation treatment, so sensitive that they can be cured by it even when secondary growths have formed. There are also some types of cancer which are very sensitive to certain chemotherapy drugs, and these particular types can be cured even when they have spread extensively. There are some cancers which are very sensitive to the balance of various hormones in the body. These cancers can remain dormant for long periods of time if the hormone balance is changed (by taking pills or injections or by removing the glands which produce certain hormones). I will be discussing these treatments and the particular types of cancer against which they are effective in later chapters.

Limitations to Different Methods of Treating Cancer

The fact that there are so many different types of cancer is one reason why there is no treatment which cures all types of cancer. There is a second reason. Cancer cells are *not different enough* from our normal cells. After all, they are actually part of us, they are cells which belong to our bodies. Their structure is very similar to non-cancer cells. Their metabolism—internal bio-chemical processes—are very similar. They reproduce in the same way.

Remember, back in Chapter 2, we compared cancer cells with weeds in a garden? Treating cancer is like trying to get rid of weeds once they are established. As with surgical removal of cancer growths, we can just pull the weeds out. This is unlikely to get rid of them permanently because we can only pull out what we can see. We know that any seeds or roots left behind may produce more weeds in the future. In addition, if the weeds are growing close to the normal plants and have extensive root systems it is likely that we will have to pull out and damage normal plants if we are to get rid of all the weeds we can see.

What about radiation treatment? We could try exposing the weeds to blazing sun while shading the normal plants. If they are growing close together it would not be possible to avoid scorching some of the normal plants. Thus this method is also very unlikely to work without some harm to normal plants. Radiation shares another problem with surgery: both methods only deal with the weeds we can see (cancer deposits we know about). Any tiny seeds or roots lying undetected and dormant cannot be eradicated by these methods.

We could try poisoning the weeds—this would be like chemo-therapy. However, because the weeds (cancer cells) belong to the same family as the normal plants (all cells belonging to us), any weedkiller would damage the normal plants. A really successful weedkiller would attack some feature common to all the weeds but not shared by the good plants. Unfortunately no such weak point has been discovered for cancer cells. Because of this, all chemotherapy drugs have some harmful effects on normal cells (side effects). Although the chemotherapy drugs that are used damage cancer cells more than normal ones, there are none which are completely harmless for normal cells.

Some methods of cancer treatment such as meditation and prayer utilise processes about which very little is known. An exceptional person may be able to rid their garden of weeds by meditating or praying over it. Equally rarely, someone may succeed in ridding their body of cancer by these methods. I don't doubt that the mind has fantastic abilities which unfortunately remain completely unexplored and untapped by most of us in today's 'civilised' and scientific society. Very few have a natural ability to tap into these powers. It seems unlikely that the rest of us could be taught to do so over a short period of time.

What about starving the weeds by depriving them of some of the nutrients they need? Some dietary methods try to 'starve' the cancer cells, for example the 'grape diet'. Again the problem is that the normal cells need the same nutrients as the cancer cells. They are not so different that we can starve the cancer cells without starving the normal cells as well.

Diet-based cancer treatments are also said to work by cleansing and purifying the body. Contaminated soil certainly can be the reason for getting a lot of weeds in the first place. However, purifying the soil in some way *after* the weeds are established seems unlikely to get rid of them. Once established, they are likely to flourish in any soil that suits their close relatives, the normal plants. 'Cleansing' the body may prevent cancer but seems unlikely to cure established cancer.

In summary, the basic fact that prevents treatments from curing all cancers is that the cancer cells are *too similar* to our normal body cells. This fact also means that no effective cancer treatment is completely free of side effects—unwanted effects in the form of damage to normal cells and parts of the body.

WEIGHING 'COST' AGAINST 'BENEFIT' WHEN CHOOSING TREATMENT

This leads me to a very important point—*for every successful cancer treatment a price must be paid.* Some treatments are much more 'costly' than others, some are much more effective than others. What is important is the balance between 'cost' and effectiveness. To judge the possible cost you need to know about the nature and likelihood of any inconvenience, disruption to normal lifestyle and side effects. To judge the possible benefits you need to know both the aim of the treatment—whether control of symptoms of cancer, temporary control of the cancer or permanent cure—and what the chances are of achieving that aim. You need to weigh the nature and chance of possible 'success' against the possible cost. If there is considerable possible benefit, you may think a considerable cost is justified. For little benefit you would probably not be prepared to pay a great 'price'. You cannot assess any treatment without knowing *both sides of this balance*—the likely cost and the likely benefit.

I use the word 'likely' because, of course, no one can ever look into the future and tell you exactly what will happen to you as an individual. You have to use probabilities and not certainties when weighing up the balance of cost versus benefit. This balance must be considered for each possible treatment. Always remember to include treatment of symptoms only (with no actual anti-cancer treatment) as one of the alternatives to assess. This alternative will not always be mentioned by your practitioner, so it is easy to forget. Where the recommended anti-cancer treatments are very heavy in cost and very light in likely benefit, the decision to have no anti-cancer treatment at all may well be the best and bravest decision you could make.

This concept of balancing cost against benefit is very important. Try to keep it in mind as you read on.

HOW YOUR DOCTOR DECIDES WHAT TREATMENT TO RECOMMEND AND WHAT THIS MEANS FOR YOU

I think many people believe that the 'experts' weigh up such a balance on their behalf. You might imagine that the treatment your practitioner recommends is based on a careful assessment, considering all aspects of each possible treatment as well as your personal, social and psychological situation and needs. That is far from the truth. Below I describe how most practitioners really decide what treatment is best. Firstly, they consider only the sorts of treatment they themselves believe in. What they believe in is determined by their training and personal attitudes.

CHOOSING YOUR TREATMENT

Best for Doctor may not be Best for You

Modern cancer specialists believe in scientifically-tested treatments which work in a way that makes sense to their scientifically-trained minds. The 'best' treatments are those which have been scientifically shown to produce the greatest proportion of remissions and the greatest average length of life, almost regardless of any other consideration. The 'best' treatments are those that are best at shrinking cancers and delaying death. They are *not* the treatments that make people *feel* best, nor are they the treatments that are most convenient and pleasant. A treatment which has any chance at all, however small, of temporarily making cancer growths smaller is 'better' than treatment aimed at simply relieving symptoms and making people *feel* better. A treatment which, on average, extends patients lives by three months is 'better' than no anti-cancer treatment. These treatments are considered better even though they may mean frequent injections, blood tests, hospital visits, weakness, nausea and vomiting and other unpleasant side effects. Doctors have set recommendations for each type of cancer. All that your doctor needs to know about *you* is the type of cancer you have, its extent and possibly your age. The same sorts of statements could be made about practitioners other than doctors.

Thus practitioners do not weigh cost against benefit when recommending treatments. They barely consider cost. The only benefits they usually believe to be important are those to do with size of tumours and length of life.

What I have said so far you probably recognise to be true, not because it agrees with what you have been taught but because it agrees with your own experience. If so, you may have already realised that the 'best' treatment in the eyes of the doctor is often not the best treatment in the eyes of the person with cancer. Unfortunately, doctors rarely allow patients to come to their own conclusions as to the best treatment. They don't offer alternatives, they don't give basic information, often they don't even justify their own treatment advice. Basically most doctors treat people with cancer like dependent children.

Like many fathers, doctors are used to being in a position of power and authority. They want their patients (children) to be obedient and submissive. They are used to telling patients what to do and they are used to patients meekly obeying their instructions. To share basic information and explain and justify their own decisions would be to weaken their power and to undermine their authority. Patients who ask questions are often treated like naughty and rebellious children. How do fathers deal with children who threaten their authority? They get angry. Or they act as though they are too busy and/or important to bother with answering such silly questions. Or they simply ignore the questions. Or they answer using words that are beyond the child's understanding, hoping to embarass them out of asking any more questions. Or they dismiss the questions with a fatherly pat on the shoulder and a patronising statement such as: 'Just leave it all to me' or 'I'll take care of you' or 'I know what's best for you'. Do you recognise these tactics? Many doctors use them to establish and maintain a paternalistic type of control over their patients.

Don't let your doctor treat you like this. You are a responsible adult and you deserve to be treated like one. It is *your* cancer, *your* comfort and *your* life that's at stake. You can make better decisions for yourself than anybody else can. Don't let anyone bully or cajole you out of your basic right to be in control of what happens to your own body.

Letting the Experts Decide?

In case you still believe that experts always make better decisions than you could, here are some actual examples of what can and does happen. Some surgeons do pointless extensive and mutilating operations to remove *secondary* growths. Doctors often recommend intensive chemotherapy to patients with cancers for which it makes no difference to the average length of life. The only 'benefit' is that the growths of a minority of patients get smaller for a short time. Thus, chemotherapy is often recommended when it has only, say, a one in twenty chance of temporarily (for a few weeks or months) shrinking cancer growths and no chance at all of curing the cancer. Doctors sometimes continue patients on chemotherapy while their cancer growths are actually getting bigger and more extensive. Practitioners whose patients' cancers continue to grow while undergoing treatment with cleansing diets usually still exhort them to persevere with their diets and take no medications at all, not even painkillers.

I am saying that many practitioners who specialise in treating cancer routinely advise unpleasant treatment that is unlikely to produce any substantial benefit *and* that they persist in recommending various anti-cancer treatments right to the bitter end. These practitioners seem unable to recognise any point when the possible benefit *for the person with cancer* is too small to justify the 'cost' *for the person with cancer* of starting or continuing further treatment. I emphasise the words 'for the person with cancer' because I believe this is the key to understanding this behaviour. And let's face it—the sorts of behaviour I have described could seem crazy to any observer with a bit of commonsense who knows what the treatments involve and how unlikely they are to produce any real benefit.

I believe the basic problem is that these practitioners do *not* act according to what is best for their individual patients. They behave like a conceited general whose soldiers are people with cancer, whose weapons are anti-cancer treatments and whose enemies are cancer and death. The general can observe the battles from a safe vantage point on a nearby mountain top. His aim is to win the battle, not to do what is best for his individual soldiers. Even when the odds are overwhelming and defeat certain, he refuses to give the order to surrender. The soldiers are not kept informed of the stage the battle is at nor given the opportunity to decide for themselves to surrender. The general will not order a surrender because this would mean admitting to his soldiers and to himself that he is not all-powerful and that he cannot control the enemy. He would rather that his soldiers die in battle than that they realise that there are limits to his power.

Some practitioners are simply unable to tell their patients that control of their cancer is beyond the practitioner's power. To advise not having, or stopping, anti-cancer treatment would be to admit that this is so. Thus these practitioners keep on recommending highly potent and unpleasant treatments when they are either known to be extremely unlikely to do any good or are experimental. Or course, these practitioners justify their actions to themselves, their colleagues and the patient's relatives. When questioned they say: 'I can't tell that patient that I can do nothing because that would be cruel—it would take all hope away.' This sort of statement actually confirms my claim that these practitioners are solely concerned with fighting cancer, not with treating whole people. When there is no effective anti-cancer treatment available, they say they can do *nothing*. When there is no hope of curing the cancer they say that stopping treatment would take all hope away. Practitioners who care for whole people would never think or say that they can do nothing. They know that treating symptoms, giving time, care, reassurance and a sympathetic ear are all doing something! Practitioners who care for whole people know that cure of their cancer is not the only thing that patients hope for. They recognise and try to fulfill other hopes—hopes for relief of pain, for time to spend at home with family and loved ones, for realistic information that will allow time for goodbyes and grieving.

Of course, not all doctors and other practitioners who treat cancer are as black as I have painted. I hope that your practitioners combine the best of modern scientific medicine with the art of healing. I hope they take as much care in finding out how you are feeling and what life is like for you as they do in arranging and assessing tests. I hope your practitioners place as much, or more, importance on the quality of your life as they do on its length. I hope they treat you as a whole person who happens to have cancer and not just as a cancer with a body wrapped around it!

If you don't have this kind of practitioner, life is going to be difficult for you. Those practitioners who are least likely to make the best decisions for you are also the most difficult to get enough information from to make your own decisions. Switch to another practitioner, if possible. If not, you may have to seek information from other sources such as other practitioners, nurses, other hospital staff, books, other patients, and friends. If you make a decision that does not follow such a practitioner's recommend-ation, be prepared to be told by them that you are foolish, ignorant and incapable of properly assessing the situation. Trust your own judgement and commonsense. Don't be intimidated or cajoled into giving away control of what happens to your own body. Remember, you are the world's greatest expert on yourself. Nobody else knows how you feel inside and what is important for you. This personal knowledge is of vital importance when it comes to deciding on treatment that could totally alter your life.

WHY YOU ARE THE BEST PERSON TO MAKE DECISIONS ABOUT YOUR OWN TREATMENT

However good and caring your practitioner is, he or she can only consider the medical side of things when recommending treatment. *You* are the *only* person who can combine the facts about possible treatments with your own 'inside' knowledge in order to arrive at the best decision for you. You know whether it is important for you to live as long as possible whatever the cost. You know how important the changes in lifestyle likely to result from your disease or treatment are to you. You know how important your body image is to you and what things about it are most important for you. Provided you can get the necessary 'outside' information, this all makes you, without question, the best person to make the decisions.

I'll just mention one thing that makes these decisions difficult for anyone, not just for you. Nobody can look into the future and predict definitely what will happen to you, as an individual, if you take a particular course of action. Your practitioner should be able to tell you what is average or likely, what is possible but unlikely and what is so unlikely as to be a miracle if it happens. To start with you should base your decision on what is likely. All patients hope they'll be the exception—the one who makes a miraculous recovery. By all means keep hoping for this, but base your decisions realistically on what is likely or average. Say your practitioner tells you that one in ten patients get a remission on a particular treatment—that means that nine in ten patients do not. If you have this treatment, you are not likely to get a remission.

Say your practitioner tells you that, on a certain treatment, half the patients live six months or less, but one in twenty live for more than two years. This means that if you have this treatment you will probably not live much longer than six months and you are very unlikely to live for more than two years. You will not make the best decisions for yourself if you base them on the hope that you will be the exception.

Although you only know what is *likely* to start with, it doesn't stay that way. As time passes, you and your practitioner find out what actually *does* happen to you. Therefore be prepared to review your decisions as time goes by. For example, say you decided with the help of your practitioner to start on a course of chemotherapy treatment. Before starting you knew there was a certain chance of experiencing particular side effects, of symptoms of the disease being helped, of the cancer going into remission and so on. Within a few days or weeks of starting treatment you actually experience certain side effects of treatment. Within a few weeks or months of starting treatment you actually discover whether or not your cancer is responsive to the treatment. As these developments actually occur, your treatment should be reviewed. For example, doses could be altered, means of controlling side effects added, different chemotherapy drugs substituted, chemotherapy stopped altogether and so on. Decisions about treatment (and indeed about most things) are not fixed or binding. The need to modify treatment as time goes by does not mean the wrong decision was made in the first place. Initial decisions are made on the basis of probabilities, later decisions can be made on the basis of actual individual facts.

Your inside knowledge is just as important with these ongoing modifications to treatment as it was with the initial decision. Your practitioner may advise you to continue intensive chemotherapy because the secondary deposits on your chest X-ray have stopped growing since starting treatment. This means that the cancer has stopped getting bigger, but has not actually got smaller. That is one important piece of information. You also know how you feel inside, how much your usual lifestyle has changed, whether the symptoms due to the cancer have improved, whether or not side effects of treatment are preventing you from doing things that are important for you. Consider *all* of the facts that have unfolded with the passage of time—not just the ones that are obvious to your practitioner. You may or may not come to the same conclusion as to the best course of action to follow.

CANCER TREATMENT RESEARCH

Testing New Treatments

Many cancer patients are involved in research into cancer treatment. It is important for you to understand something about this. In Great Britain, the approval of an ethical committee is necessary before any trials can proceed involving patients. These committees should have a non-medical member who is supposed to evaluate the research proposal from the patients' point of view. The committees are sometimes asked to consider trials in which the patient is not informed of their participation—and cannot therefore give consent. Basically, there are three different stages of testing for new treatments.

Phase I Studies

In Phase I studies, researchers test drugs or other treatments that have never before been tried on humans. They have been tested only in the laboratory and on various animals. As well as testing for the drug's anti-cancer properties, Phase I studies are designed to find out how the treatment can be used in humans. The aim is to find out things such as whether it can be taken by mouth or injection, whether it is broken down by the liver or passed out through the kidneys, what doses are safe, how often they should be given and what side effects there are. Because these things are not known, patients in these tests may experience unexpected and unpleasant side effects as a result of the treatment. Therefore, only patients for whom there is no known effective anti-cancer treatment available are asked to take part in these studies. You might be happy to participate, knowing that by doing so you could help future patients. However, if you go into it because you hope it will help you personally, you might well be disappointed.

Phase II Studies

In Phase II studies, the aim is to find out what human cancers are sensitive to the new treatment. Although these tests are not usually as unpleasant and dangerous, again only patients who have already had all known effective anti-cancer treatments are asked to take part. Researchers are now mainly trying to find out about effects against cancer, so they concentrate on measuring size of cancer growths. If some patients' growths do get smaller, further testing is carried out on their particular types of cancer in Phase III studies (see below). If none of the first fourteen patients with a certain type of cancer show any reduction in their tumours, the treatment is not usually tested any further.

Again, if your main reason for agreeing to be a research subject is the hope that it will benefit you personally, you might be disappointed.

Phase III Studies

Treatments that are found to be active against certain types of cancer are then further tested in Phase III studies. In this phase of research, the aim is to find out whether the new treatment is better than what is already available. Not only completely new treatments but also variations on old treatments are tested—for example, different combinations, dosages or timing of previously available drugs.

No sophisticated research or statistical methods would be necessary if we were looking only for major improvements in treatment. It is a fact that the greatest advances in cancer treatment have been made simply by trying a completely new type of treatment in a series of patients. Here are some examples concerning chemotherapy.

How Major Improvements In Chemotherapy Have Come About

Prior to the early 1960s, chemotherapy was in its infancy and the drugs were used one at a time. A few types of cancer were found to be very sensitive to particular drugs. Some cancers were even cured—for example, the rare cancer of women called chorio-carcinoma could be completely cured by the drug methotrexate. As there was previously no effective treatment for these cancers, it was very obvious that the new treatment was a major improvement!

In the early 1960s, a group of doctors from the United States reported using a revolutionary new technique. They combined high doses of four different chemotherapy drugs (mustine, vincristine, procarbazine and prednisone) to produce a treatment that produced remissions in the majority of patients with Hodgkin's disease. Prior to this, extensive Hodgkin's disease was fatal within a few months. Now patients were living for years and, in fact, many of them later proved to be completely cured. The improvement in results was so great and significant that no special research techniques were needed to prove it.

In the mid-1970s, the same degree of improvement occurred in the treatment of testicular cancer. This time it was a new drug rather than a new technique (the use of high dose combinations) that was responsible for the breakthrough. A new drug called cis-platinum had been shown to be active against testicular cancer in Phase II studies. This drug, when combined with the two previously best drugs (vinblastine and bleomycin) produced complete remissions in most patients with cancer of the testes, many of whom were later shown to be cured altogether. Prior to that about one in three patients with extensive cancer of the testes experienced remissions which were only partial and temporary, cures were unusual. Again, special research techniques were not necessary to prove that the new treatment was much better than what had been used previously.

Unfortunately, dramatic and obvious improvements in treatment like these are rare. After the results in Hodgkin's disease were published, the principle of using high dose combinations was applied to other types of cancer. A few types showed a similarly dramatic improvement in results but for many it was much less spectacular or nonexistent. For example, about one in three people with extensive breast cancer gain a remission with single chemotherapy drug treatment and their average length of life is about nine months. About two in three people get remissions with combination chemotherapy and their average length of life is about twenty-one months, none are completely cured. In cancer of the large bowel and most types of lung cancer, no combinations of drugs result in people living any longer, on average, than those who have no anti-cancer treatment at all. Combinations using the drug cis-platinum are far less effective against other types of cancer than they are against testicular cancer.

Unfortunately, it is a fact that dramatic breakthroughs in treatment are rare and usually only apply to a few particular types of cancer. In testing most new treatments, cancer specialists are looking for differences that are 'statistically significant', that is unlikely to be due to chance, rather than dramatic breakthroughs which would be self-evident. 'Statistically significant' does *not* mean significant for large numbers of people, as you will see.

Randomised Clinical Trials

The main technique used in this endeavour is the randomised clinical trial. Here doctors select a fairly uniform group of people — all within a certain age range, with similar types and extent of cancer and about the same degree of physical fitness. To further reduce any possible bias, the people in this already fairly uniform group are allotted *randomly* (by chance) to one or other of the treatments to be compared. Doctors believe that such random allocation of people to treatment is the best way of making sure that any differences in results are due to the different treatments and not to any other factor. As I have explained, such techniques are only necessary if we are looking for small differences. For example, trials often include *hundreds* of people in an attempt to make sure that they do not miss differences of five per cent (one in twenty) in remission rates or of a few weeks or months in average length of life. These are regarded as 'statistically significant' differences. The researchers are looking for results that can be accurately measured and subjected to statistical analysis—things like remission rate and length of life.

How important are these statistically significant differences to patients? This is a question that some doctors forget to ask themselves or to allow their patients to decide. I have heard doctors claim that a treatment involving five different injections which caused nausea, low blood counts, hair loss and many other unpleasant side effects was 'better' than a treatment consisting only of tablets with very few side effects. The first treatment was 'better' because it produced a statistically significant improvement in the average length of life—three months longer than with the tablets. So when your doctor recommends a certain treatment, telling you that research has shown it to be the 'best', make sure you find out just what this means and what the alternatives are. Given *all* the information about each treatment, you may or may not agree with your doctor's conclusion.

Importance of Clinical Trials for You

Clinical trials are important to you in two ways. Firstly, results from them are used by doctors to determine which treatment is 'best'. Secondly, you may be asked to take part in them. An important aspect of clinical trials for you—the person with cancer—is that if you agree to take part in them you obviously don't get to decide on your own treatment (and nor, incidentally, does your doctor, because the treatment is decided by chance). You would be asked to agree to be *randomised* and then to have whichever treatment you are allotted by chance. Taking part in this type of clinical trial is not necessarily of any benefit to you personally. Also it may be of little benefit to future patients because such small differences between treatments are being looked for. If people with cancer were given the choice between treatments, they might place more importance on things like convenience, side effects, comfort and time in hospital than on whether or not one or the other is likely to produce a few extra weeks or months of life.

Your Rights Regarding Clinical Trials

Don't forget that you have the right to refuse to take part in clinical trials. If you do agree, you have the right to withdraw at any stage simply because you don't want to keep having the randomly allotted treatment—you don't need any more reason than that. If you refuse from the start or withdraw later, your doctors are obliged to continue to treat you to the best of their ability and without prejudice. If you know or suspect they are not doing this, it would be best to switch to another doctor, if this is possible.

As you know, your informed consent (written) is necessary before you can be treated in any form of research trial. I know that, definitely in Australia, and possibly in other countries, some patients are treated in clinical trials without their knowledge or consent. Some doctors randomise their patients and *then* tell them that they recommend the treatment to which they have in fact already been allotted by chance. The only way you could suspect this is happening is if your doctor is particularly adamant that you follow his or her recommendation (although of course this may simply be a reaction to the fact that your questioning is undermining your doctor's authority). You should ask directly if you suspect that you are being treated in a research project without your consent.

DEFINITIONS OF SOME EXPRESSIONS YOUR DOCTOR MAY USE

Expressions Used To Describe Aims Of Treatment

Potentially Curative Treatment

Potentially curative treatment, or treatment with curative intent, are truthful expressions that are sometimes incorrectly shortened to 'curative treatment'. This last term wrongly implies that all patients having the treatment will be cured. **Potentially curative** treatment is treatment that is capable of completely and permanently curing a cancer. Some potentially curative treatments actually do cure most of the patients having them, others cure only a small proportion. If your doctor tells you that a proposed treatment is potentially curative, make sure you find out what the *chance* of cure by it is. You need to know this to weigh up the benefit against the cost. If there is only a five per cent (one in twenty) chance of cure you might be less prepared to accept its cost than if it is a ninety-five per cent (nineteen in twenty).

Remember that we can only know that a treatment is potentially curative if it has been in use for many years. If your practitioner says he or she can cure you with a treatment that has only been in use for a few months or years, *don't believe them*. It's that simple. It could be true that immediately after completing the treatment there are indeed some patients in whom no cancer can be detected by currently available tests. However, as you already know from earlier chapters in this book, this does not necessarily mean that no cancer cells at all are left. Remember, there are no tests currently available that can pick up very tiny seedlings. We can only say that patients have been completely cured in retrospect, that is, after enough time has gone by for any remaining tiny seedlings to activate and form obvious secondary growths. This time is different for different types of cancer, but is never less than two years. Usually it is from five to twenty or more years.

Palliative and Symptomatic Treatments

Palliative treatment is treatment that has *no* chance of permanently curing you. Your doctor knows from the start whether proposed treatments are potentially curative or palliative. Insist that you know too. Most patients are prepared to accept very much greater costs for potentially curative treatment than for palliative treatment. Palliative treatment used to always mean treatment aimed at making patients feel better. This sort of palliative treatment is also called **symptomatic** treatment because it is aimed at relief of symptoms. Symptoms are the effects of your disease or treatment that make you feel uncomfortable — things such as pain, nausea, coughing, breathlessness, diarrhoea, mouth ulcers, bleeding and so on. Thus symptomatic treatment means things like pain-killers, anti-nausea treatment, oxygen, cough suppressants, removal of pleural fluid, transfusions, mouth washes and so on. Symptomatic treatment is always very important for you. However, some doctors concentrate so hard on treating the cancer, that they neglect to pay enough attention to your symptoms. They can and should be treated, whether or not you are also having anti-cancer treatment. Tell your doctor what symptoms you are having and insist that something be done about them.

Nowadays, the term palliative treatment also includes treatments aimed at temporarily controlling the cancer itself. Such treatment can include surgery, radiotherapy, chemotherapy and other anti-cancer treatments. We have already seen that this approach does not necessarily result in patients *feeling* better, in fact it often makes them feel worse.

Possible Benefits of Palliative Treatment

The possible benefit of palliative anti-cancer treatments is that they *may* control the cancer *temporarily*. While the cancer is under control, there will probably be less symptoms from it. The patient *may* feel better, provided the symptoms due to treatment are not as bad as the symptoms due to the cancer were. Sooner or later the cancer will become active again. It will then grow and eventually result in death in much the same way as it would have earlier, if no anti-cancer treatment had been used. In other words, the possible benefit from palliative cancer treatments is that they may *delay* the eventual outcome. However, they don't really *alter* it. In contrast, potentially curative treatments may prevent a person from dying *of cancer*. Try not to lose sight of the fact that, of course, there is nothing that can prevent you from eventually dying *of something*. A lot of people with cancer suffer unnecessarily because they let their doctors treat them as though this was not a basic fact of life.

Know the Aim of Your Treatment

Many patients also suffer unnecessarily because they don't know the actual aim of their treatment. It is a sad but true fact that many patients have palliative anti-cancer treatments believing they may be cured by them. Many doctors do not make the aim of treatment clear to their patients. Quite often, doctors recommend very extensive surgery or potent chemotherapy with a lot of side effects to people with cancers that cannot be cured. Most of these people wrongly take it for granted that such severe treatments would only be recommended if they had a chance of curing them. Make sure *you* know exactly what can be achieved by any proposed treatment. You may have to ask directly, and more than once, to get a straight answer.

Expressions Used To Describe Effects Of Treatment

Remissions—Complete and Partial

The word **remission** means that the cancer growths have got smaller. If your doctor tells you that you are in a **complete remission**, this is certainly extremely good news. It means that no traces of cancer can be found in your body at that particular time. It does *not* guarantee that there are no cancer cells still in your body. As you already know, there are no tests that can detect very tiny cancer seedlings. Fair enough, you may say, but surely a complete remission means at least a definite *possibility* of permanent cure. I'm afraid that even this is not always true. Complete remissions can be produced by palliative cancer treatments. These remissions are never permanent. On the other hand, a complete remission with potentially curative treatment certainly does mean *possible* permanent cure. You can't say it is a *definite* cure until later—after enough years have gone by for any dormant seedlings to activate and make their presence obvious.

The expression **partial remission** means the cancer deposits have got smaller, but are still detectable. They can still be felt, or seen on X-rays, scans, biopsies etc, or detected through blood tests. A treatment that quickly produces a partial remission may eventually produce a complete remission if continued. People with partial remissions tend to live longer than people whose cancers don't respond to treatment. However, of course, no one who has only a partial remission is ever cured.

Stable Disease

Your doctor may tell you that you have **stable disease**. This means that the cancer has not changed in size since you started treatment—it hasn't got bigger but it hasn't got smaller either. It is most unlikely that continuing this treatment will bring you any real advantage. You would just be experiencing the side effects of treatment for no benefit other than *perhaps* living slightly longer.

Relapse or Recurrence

A **relapse** or **recurrence** means that the cancer is growing again after a period of being dormant. If you were in partial remission, the growths, which had temporarily got smaller but not disappeared, have started to grow again. If you were in complete remission, and have now relapsed, this means that tiny seedlings were actually there all along. They have now reactivated and grown to a size that is detectable. The **remission duration** or length of remission is the time between diagnosis of remission and diagnosis of relapse.

The seriousness of a relapse depends on your type of cancer and what previous treatment you have had. If you have a type of cancer for which radiotherapy or chemotherapy is potentially curative and if you have previously been treated only by surgery, you could still be cured completely. If you have one of these types of cancer but have already been treated with chemotherapy or radiotherapy, it is very unlikely that you would be cured by using the same treatment again. Usually, a temporary remission would be the most that you could realistically hope for. The first remission is the easiest to achieve, lasts the longest and is really the only one that could eventually prove to be a cure. Unless a completely different form of treatment is used, second remissions are harder to achieve, last a shorter time and very rarely prove to be complete cures. Bear this in mind if your doctor recommends treatment for a relapse.

What You Need to Know to Make the Best Decisions

Now we come to the question which hangs on every patient's lips, although some never dare to actually ask it: 'How long will I live?'

Many patients avoid asking this question because they fear the answer so much. In my experience, most patients actually imagine that things are *worse* than they really are. Thus the answer may come as a pleasant surprise. Whether or not this is so for you, I believe it is always easier to deal with facts than with the products of your imagination. In any case, you cannot possibly make the best decisions for yourself if you don't know what difference various treatments are likely to make to the length of your life.

This question is also hard to answer, partly because no one can look into the future and tell you exactly what will happen to you as an individual. Many doctors use this as an excuse to avoid giving any answer at all. However, they *can* tell you what is average or likely, what is possible but unlikely and what is so unlikely as to be a miracle if it happens. I believe that the following is the least you need to find out from your doctor in order to make the best possible decision about treatment. Firstly, is it possible that any treatment could completely cure you, that is, that you could live as long as if you hadn't ever had the cancer? Secondly, what is the median length of life for each possible anti-cancer treatment, and also if you have no anti-cancer treatment at all? The **median** (or average) length of life is the time between diagnosis or starting treatment and when half of the patients have died. Thirdly, what is the chance that you could live for five years? (This is called the five year survival time.)

Say your doctor tells you that one in twenty (five per cent) of patients with your particular type and stage of cancer are cured with a particular treatment. The median survival is twelve months. The five year survival is one in twenty (five per cent). What does this mean for you? It means that if you have this treatment, there is a fifty-fifty chance that you will live less than twelve months. There is only a one in twenty chance that you will live five years but if you do, you will know you are almost certainly completely cured. Imagine for the same situation, if your doctor simply said 'You *could* be completely cured and live as long as you would have if you had never had the cancer'. This is true but doesn't really give a complete picture. A patient told only this would be much more likely to agree to a twelve month course of intensive chemotherapy than a patient who knew that there was a fifty per cent chance of dying before even completing the treatment. So do make sure that you get more detailed information than what is possible but unlikely. This is the part the doctor is most likely to tell you, but on its own and without percentage figures it can be very misleading.

What can we conclude now? You have cancer and that is bad news, whichever way you look at it. There are probably difficult times ahead of you, whatever you do. If you meekly accept all your practitioner's recommendations, it is likely that life will be much less pleasant for you than it could be. If you try to make your own decisions, it is likely that you will have difficulty getting the cooperation and information you need from your practitioner. Seek support from family, friends, nurses, social workers, or other practitioners. Trust your own judgement and gut feelings about what is right for you. Don't let your practitioner talk you out of your decisions with medical jargon, scientific explanations, bullying or sweet-talking. These are techniques that authority figures such as fathers and teachers use with children. Switch to a practitioner who doesn't do this, if possible. If not, just remember that you are not a child and that they can only hold a position of power and authority over you if you let them.

Here is a thought that might help you a little. Every time you refuse to let a practitioner treat you like a helpless child, you make it that tiny bit easier for the next patient to do the same. It is only through pressure from patients like you that doctors and other practitioners will be forced to change their approach. I believe this is the most important way in which you can use your disease to help future patients.

Chapter 6

TREATMENT OF SYMPTOMS

Symptoms are what you *feel*— things such as pain, nausea, lack of energy and breathlessness. In this chapter we will talk about how to tackle symptoms that worry you for any reason.

Of course, now that you have cancer, I know that *every* symptom you get will worry you to start with. You probably feel a stab of panic whenever you notice any minor discomfort in your body because this could signal that your cancer is active. This reaction is natural and normal.

I suggest that whenever you get any new symptoms, you stop and ask yourself these questions:
- Is this symptom one that I would have worried about before I had the cancer?
- Would I have contacted my practitioner about it?
- Is there a commonsense explanation for it?
  (For example, unusual activity that could have caused muscle pains, something you ate that could have caused nausea or indigestion, tension that could have caused a headache.)

The answers to these question will help you to decide what action you should take. For example, if you would have waited a few days to see how it went before you had cancer, that's probably still what you should do. If you would have accepted a commonsense explanation for it before, you probably should now. The symptoms that still worry you after this sort of check are the ones that will mainly concern us in this chapter.

I'm afraid that many doctors and other practitioners who treat people with cancer behave as though symptoms are not important. These practitioners don't ask about them and will treat you in an inattentive and impatient manner if you try to tell them about the symptoms that are worrying you.

You will have to keep reminding yourself of three things in order to get your symptoms the attention they deserve. Firstly, any symptom that is uncomfortable, restricts your activity, keeps you awake, makes you feel anxious because you don't know what it means or worries you in any other way, *is* important. Secondly, because no one else can see or feel your symptoms, they will only know about them if you tell them. Thirdly, your practitioner's job is to care for you as a whole person, not just to treat your cancer. It is never a waste of his or her time to talk about your symptoms. In fact, your symptoms and their treatment should be discussed every time you see your practitioner.

What if your practitioner refuses to pay attention to your symptoms and behaves as though tests and anti-cancer treatments are more important than your comfort? In this case, I suggest you very seriously consider changing practitioners. This will be easiest for those of you who are not having any specialised treatment. If you are, it may still be possible to find a practitioner who can both supervise your specialised treatment and take care of *you*. If you can't find such a person, you could consider continuing the specialised treatment under your original expert's supervision, while seeing another practitioner for care of your symptoms. Your local general practitioner may be prepared and able to do this.

Yet another possibility is to stop your specialised treatment. Think carefully about the costs and benefits of continuing with it. To the costs you considered when agreeing to have it, you must now add the fact that your symptoms are being ignored. As a result, you are experiencing discomfort and inconvenience. This extra cost could be enough to tip the balance in favour of stopping your treatment.

Tackling Your Symptoms

How *should* your symptoms be tackled? Firstly, your practitioner should listen to your description. Next he or she should ask questions to help find out how much they are worrying, disabling or otherwise inconveniencing you, and to establish their cause. It is important that neither you nor your practitioner jump to the conclusion that your cancer is the cause for every symptom you get. Just as it was before you had cancer, the cause for any symptom must be looked for. To this end, your practitioner may need to examine you and arrange tests.

Next your practitioner should advise you on treatment for the symptoms. They can be treated either by tackling them directly or by treating their cause or both. For example, the pain of a broken leg can be treated with painkillers or by setting the fracture and immobilising the leg in a plaster cast, or both.

As a rule, treating the cause brings more long-lasting benefits than just treating the symptom itself. However, even if cancer is the cause of your symptoms, this does not mean that treating the cancer is necessarily the best approach. As always, you will have to weigh the cost against the benefit to decide what is best.

Staying at Home or Going Into Hospital

There is *no* symptom that automatically means you have to go into hospital. However, you may choose to go into hospital for tests or to have some form of treatment that cannot be done at home. The need for hospitalisation is one of the costs you should take into account when deciding what tests and treatment to have.

The decision as to whether to stay at home or go into hospital in the final stages should largely be yours. However, a decision to stay at home is practical only if you can rely on a lot of support and cooperation from family and friends. I suggest that, if you do want to be at home, you make some preparations towards this while you are still relatively well. Talk with your family and friends about what you want and find out how much help and support they are prepared and able to give you. Get to know a doctor who will make home visits. Find out whether there is a special palliative care/terminal care/hospice team in your town and ask to be referred to them when the time seems right for that. Your doctor can arrange for a district nurse, or a Macmillan nurse or a nurse from the Marie Curie Foundation who specialise in care for cancer patients, to visit you at home for a particular purpose such as to do dressings, supervise pressure care, help you with bowel or bladder problems or just for a friendly check on how you are managing. Special aids that you might need such as wheelchairs, bedpans, commodes, special bedding, oxygen masks, etc, are often available on loan from hospitals or through the home nursing services, so the fact that you can't afford to buy such things shouldn't mean that you have to go into hospital.

You may also be able to get financial assistance from the social services, for example you can claim Attendance Allowance if you need a lot of help from another person.

Symptoms and Nervous Tension

Everybody who has cancer is under some nervous strain some of the time. This shows itself in different ways in different people. Symptoms which can be due to nervous tension include difficulty sleeping, lack of energy, irritability, crying spells, loss of appetite, nausea, difficulty in swallowing, indigestion, stomach pains, diarrhoea, breathlessness, chest pains, palpitations, headache, neck pain and many others. Each of these symptoms can also have other causes. For example, nausea may be due to anxiety, but may also be due to cancer in the stomach, liver or brain, to chemotherapy, radiotherapy, stomach ulcers, a hangover, viruses, excessive calcium in the blood and so on.

It can sometimes be quite difficult to work out which factors are playing a part in producing a certain symptom. Often it is more than one. It is not unusual for symptoms that begin for a physical reason to be aggravated by nervous tension. For instance, anxiety about nausea with chemotherapy can aggravate it and even result in it starting *before* you have your injection or tablets.

While recognising that nervous tension can produce or aggravate physical symptoms, neither you nor your practitioner should jump to the conclusion that this is happening, without first checking other possibilities. If your practitioner dismisses a symptom as being due to nervous tension and you don't feel this conclusion is right, I suggest you ask for a second opinion.

On the other hand, if you and your practitioner come to the

conclusion that a symptom is caused or aggravated by nervous tension, this is not something to be ashamed or embarrassed about. You are under enormous strain and it would be surprising if your nerves did not play up in some way. Symptoms caused or aggravated by nervous tension are no less important, real or uncomfortable than any others. You are a whole person, not just a physical body. All parts of you are important and interconnected. Be kind to yourself—don't judge yourself harshly, but respect and take care of all of you!

Once you accept that nervous tension is playing a part in producing a symptom, it might then improve or even clear up altogether. If not, there are basically three ways of tackling the situation. You can choose any one, two or even all three.

One approach is simply to have treatment directed at the symptoms. For example, antacid for indigestion, painkillers for headaches, or sleeping pills for sleeplessness. Another is to reduce your nervous tension by taking sedatives, or anti-depressants, or by learning relaxation techniques, meditation, yoga and so on.

However, I think that the best way to get rid of any physical or mental symptoms of nervous tension is to tackle the cause directly. Stop trying to hide or deny your feelings of sadness, anger, or fear. When you try to force these natural feelings underground they are more likely to express themselves in the form of some unpleasant symptoms. So try to let them out—talk about them and allow yourself to feel them. You may be able to do this with family, friends, your practitioner, a nurse, a priest, social worker, psychologist, or psychiatrist. Choose one or more of these people that you trust and feel comfortable with.

Any or all of these approaches may reduce your discomfort and help you to take and keep control of your life. Don't let your need to appear tough and able to cope with anything prevent you from seeking relief of all your symptoms, whatever their cause.

We'll now go on to look at some of the symptoms you could experience and what you can do about them.

PAIN

This is the symptom that you probably worry about the most, even if you don't have it! Here are some facts that may surprise you. Cancer is *not* always painful, not even at the end. Cancer pain reacts to painkillers just like any other pain. When people with cancer do get pain, it is always possible to greatly relieve it, and sometimes even to get rid of it completely.

I know why you are anxious and frightened about the possibility of pain. You have read about, heard of, or known people who did have pain with cancer and whose pain was not controlled. You, yourself, may even have pain which is not being controlled right now. *It doesn't have to be that way for you.*

We *can* do something about it. The most common reason for unrelieved cancer pain is simply *ignorance* — ignorance on the part of many doctors and nurses, as well as on the part of many people with cancer. Many doctors and nurses simply don't know enough about the individual painkillers and how to use them most effectively. They don't know how small the risk of addiction is when painkillers are used simply to control pain. Sometimes they don't even know that it *is* realistic to aim for good control of cancer pain with painkillers.

So here's what we can do about it. Read this section and make sure *you* are not ignorant about pain control. You will need to understand a fair bit about the use of painkillers yourself in order to get good pain relief. You may even have to teach your doctors and nurses something! I know it is frightening to think that your doctors and nurses may not know everything, but I believe you will be best able to deal with any pain you have if you accept this possibility. Those of you who don't have this problem, whose doctors and nurses do understand how to use painkillers effectively, will probably still find this section helpful and interesting. For the rest of you, this section is absolutely essential.

If you are in a lot of pain *right now*, I suggest you ask a trusted friend or relative to read this section and help you to carry out some of my suggestions. You will have very little energy to spare until your pain is effectively treated, so ask for help.

112

Tackling the Cause of Pain Directly

Let's start at the beginning. Let's say that the cause has been checked and your pain is due to your cancer. It may be possible to tackle this cause directly, but this would not necessarily be the best approach. You will have to weigh up the costs and benefits, just as for any other treatment.

In general, radiation is the form of anti-cancer treatment most likely to control cancer pain, especially that due to secondary cancer in the bones. This may entail only a few treatments and very little side effects. Pain due to cancer in other parts of the body, especially if the growth is large, generally requires longer treatment and higher doses and, even then, radiation is less likely to result in good pain control. Ask your doctor just what your proposed treatment would involve and how likely it is to work.

Surgery is a good way of tackling a few particular types of pain due to cancer. For example, pain due to a blockage of the bowel or kidney can sometimes be relieved by removing the responsible growth or bypassing the blockage. Pain due to a fracture through cancer in a bone, can often be most quickly relieved by putting a metal pin or plate in the bone. The bone is most likely to remain pain free if this surgery is followed up by radiation treatment.

Even chemotherapy is sometimes recommended for people who have painful cancer growths. The pain will be relieved only if the growth is shrunk, so consider this method of pain relief only if you have a type of cancer which is *very* likely to be sensitive to the chemotherapy.

If you do decide to seek pain relief by tackling the responsible cancer itself, you will still need painkillers in the meantime. The fact that your pain may be relieved by radiotherapy or surgery later doesn't mean that you shouldn't be getting relief with painkillers right now. The following section is important for all of you with cancer pain— those who are having anti-cancer treatment as well as those who are not.

Some Facts About Painkillers

Here is a table telling you some facts you will need to know about painkillers.

In the first column I have listed their chemical names. If the name of your painkiller is not on this list, it is most likely because you have been given the proprietary (drug company) name and/or because it is a mixture. Ask for the chemical name(s) of your painkiller(s).

In the second column is the dose which, if taken *by mouth*, is likely to relieve the pain of a person who is just *starting* on painkillers. These doses are all of about equal strength, so you can work out what dose of another painkiller will have about the same effect if you switch from one to another. Injections are two to four times stronger than tablets or syrup of the same drug.

The third column shows how long each dose usually lasts. Remember, everybody is different. These figures are average, just to give you the general idea.

Painkiller	*Dose* (milligrams)	*Duration of Action* (hours)
Aspirin	600	4–6
Paracetamol	600	4–6
Propoxyphene*	130–260	4–6
Codeine phosphate	120	4–6
Pentazocine*	100	2–3
Pethidine*	200	2–3
Dextromoramide* (Palfium)	10	2–4
Methadone	15	4–8
Papaveretum (Omnopon)	40	3–5
Morphine	20	4–7
Diamorphine (heroin)	15	4–7

The drugs in this list which are asterixed are ones which I do not recommend for control of cancer pain, but I have included them because they are often recommended. These drugs are more likely than the other painkillers to produce side effects such as lightheadedness, difficulty in concentrating, confusion and hallucinations. They are also inconvenient to take because they last for such a short time.

I have also included one drug I have never used because it is not legally available in Australia—heroin. You will see that heroin is about the same strength, and lasts about as long as morphine. In fact, I included heroin so that you could see that there is nothing magic about it. I do not believe that legalisation of heroin would result in greatly improved pain relief for most people with cancer. What *is* more likely to achieve this is better education of doctors and nurses in the use of the painkillers already available.

I'll just comment on one thing that may surprise you. You will see from the table that just two tablets of either aspirin or paracetamol, both easily available non-prescription painkillers, are about as strong as 20 milligrams of morphine taken by mouth. Surprising but true and very useful. You don't need to rely on your doctors for supplies of painkillers as long as one of these drugs works for you and suits you. However, it is very important to know that you must not take aspirin if you are having a chemotherapy drug called methotrexate (see p 264). Aspirin is also not a safe painkiller if you have a stomach ulcer or if you bleed and bruise easily for any reason, but especially if you have a low platelet count. A problem with both aspirin and paracetamol is that it is neither safe nor pleasant to take more than about 4,000 milligrams per day of either one (that is twelve aspirin tablets of 300 milligrams each *or* eight paracetamol tablets of 500 milligrams each). Higher doses are likely to cause heavy sweating, nausea, vomiting, dizziness, confusion, and in the case of aspirin, ringing in the ears. Too much paracetamol can cause serious liver damage and too much aspirin can seriously disturb the balance of acids and minerals in the blood. This means that, *on their own*, aspirin and paracetamol are only useful as long as less than 4,000 milligrams per day is enough to control your pain. But don't worry, there is *no such limit* for the other painkillers listed.

When you check the chemical names of what is in your painkiller against the above list, you may not find one or more of the ingredients. A likely reason is that the missing ingredient is a sedative. Ask if you are not sure. If you have been prescribed a painkilling mixture that includes a sedative, I suggest you ask for a change. The sedative will just make you more sleepy and confused without doing anything for your pain. If you want to

115

have a sedative to help you relax it is better to take it separately. You will then be able to adjust your dose of painkiller according to your pain and your dose of sedative according to your degree of relaxation.

My advice is similar if you are prescribed a painkilling mixture of morphine and alcohol. If you are taking morphine in liquid form, ask whether it contains alcohol. If you want alcohol, you will probably prefer to take it separately in a form that you enjoy and in the amount that suits you, rather than mixed with your painkiller.

How to Take Painkillers

The ideal way to take any painkiller is to take a dose that completely relieves your pain and to repeat that dose every time the pain *just starts* to come back. If you are taking your painkiller by mouth or in suppository form, it will take fifteen to thirty minutes to start working. Injections work more quickly. It will then last two to six or more hours, depending on which one it is— check the table.

Doctors often recommend that you take a painkiller only 'when you need it' (whatever that means)! People who are told to do this often wait until their pain is excruciating before taking the next dose. This is a very bad way to take painkillers since, if you do this, you will never have good pain control. You will spend most of your time feeling frightened and anxious because you know that the pain is going to come back, and it will take a bigger dose to control it when it does. It is much better to work out how long it is before your pain *just starts* to come back and to take your painkiller *regularly* that often. Remember, it will take fifteen to thirty minutes after you take it before it starts to work. If you take painkillers like this you will get good, even, pain control with smaller doses of painkiller. Don't take painkillers only when you 'need' them.

In the case of the painkillers on the list other than aspirin and paracetamol, if you take the same one regularly for some weeks, you are likely to find it is not working as well, or for as long. This is normal and expected. It does *not* mean that you are getting addicted to your painkiller. What happens is that your body develops ways of getting rid of the drug more quickly. It now takes more of the painkiller to achieve the same amount in your blood. Therefore, when you find that the dose which used to control your pain no longer does so, it is quite safe, and indeed necessary, to increase your dose. The higher dose is no more dangerous and will cause no more side effects *for you* than the usual starting dose would for someone who had not been taking painkillers.

Possible Side Effects of Painkillers

If the dose you start with does not relieve your pain completely, you should gradually increase it either until it does or until you feel that the cost of the better pain relief outweighs the benefit. Possible side effects of painkillers include nausea, constipation, heavy sweating, drowsiness, lightheadedness, difficulty in concentrating, hallucinations, confusion and dizziness. Except for constipation, all of these are worst just after starting a new painkiller or increasing your dose. They tend to clear up by themselves, so it is usually worth persevering for a few days before deciding that a particular painkiller doesn't suit you.

If, even then, you cannot find a dose that relieves your pain without unpleasant side effects, you should stop taking it altogether and change to a different painkiller. The alternative would be to add a second painkiller while continuing to take unsatisfactory doses of the first. If you do this, you are likely to finish up with much more troublesome side effects for the same degree of pain relief. It is better to find the single painkiller that suits you best and take effective doses of that.

By the way, almost all painkillers cause constipation, so changing painkillers is not a good way of dealing with this problem. You will probably need to take laxatives regularly. Read pages 130–31 for other suggestions.

Aim for the balance between pain relief and side effects that's best for you. You may prefer to be completely free of pain, even if this means that you are drowsy and can't concentrate on anything. Or you may prefer to have mild pain when you move about in exchange for feeling more alert.

It is almost always possible to relieve cancer pain with painkillers taken by mouth either in tablet or liquid form. Injections should be necessary only if you are vomiting, can't swallow, or are too sleepy to take pills or syrup. An alternative to injections is suppositories. Some painkillers, for example, pentazocine, are available in this form. The painkiller is absorbed into the system through the lining of the rectum. Their big advantage over injections is that you can use them yourself at home. Another use for suppositories is as a supplement to painkillers taken by mouth. If you use a painkilling suppository last thing at night instead of your tablets or syrup, you are likely to get a longer stretch of pain-free sleep, because suppositories are longer acting.

Painkillers and Addiction

It is a fact that many painkillers are addictive. However, it is extremely rare for people who use painkillers *as painkillers* to become addicted to them. Addiction is much, much more likely to develop in people who take painkillers not for pain relief, but in order to get a lift, escape from reality or for some other such reason. If you take painkillers for pain, you will find that you can stop taking them quite easily if, and when, your pain is relieved by some other means. Provided you stop them gradually over a couple of days, the worst that will happen is that you may get some mild withdrawal symptoms such as temporary restlessness, difficulty in sleeping and a runny nose. If you get these symptoms, it does *not* mean that you *were* addicted. It just means that your body had got used to having the drug around and is now readjusting to being without it again.

I know it is not easy to overcome a fear of addiction and just allow yourself to take as much painkiller as you need. Try to rid yourself of the idea that painkillers are things that enslave you unless you constantly struggle to take them as little as possible. Who would you say is the real slave—the person who is so immobilised and preoccupied by pain that life is miserable for themselves and their family and friends or the one who takes enough painkillers to stay relaxed and comfortable? Uncontrolled pain is a much greater tyrant than painkillers taken so that they do relieve pain.

People often voice the fear that if they take strong painkillers now, they won't work later. This is not true. There is no quota on painkillers that can leave you with nothing to fall back on once you've 'used it up'. They *will* keep working. Admittedly, as I've already mentioned, you may need a bigger dose to get the same effect, but you *can* still get the same effect. So take the painkillers you need now, they will still work later.

Sometimes people are very reluctant to take a drug such as morphine because they think this is used only in the terminal stages. This is also not true. I recommended morphine often, to people with all stages of cancer, because it is a good painkiller. People who did indeed have incurable cancer often continued to take it with good effect, for many months. Don't save strong painkillers for 'the end', use them when you need them.

Another reason you might have for taking insufficient painkillers to completely relieve pain is because you fear actual or anticipated side effects. We talked a bit about the actual side effects earlier, and the need to find the balance between pain relief and side effects that is best for you. There are also the invisible, possible future side effects like kidney damage. This is only a concern for people taking a lot of painkillers every day for *many* years, so it is not a real worry for you. Either you will recover from your cancer, in which case you won't need to keep taking painkillers or your cancer will not be cured, in which case possible kidney damage years hence is not really a concern. Either way, there's no need to let this stop you from taking the painkillers you need now.

Other Ways of Reducing Your Pain

I believe that the effective use of painkillers is absolutely central to good pain control and that is why I have discussed this first. However, there are other ways of reducing your pain which you may also want to use. Choose the combination of painkillers and other approaches that gives *you* the greatest benefit for the least cost. For example, you can experiment to find the positions for sitting and lying that are most comfortable for you. You can try to avoid activities that aggravate your pain and to get plenty of rest. Heat on the painful spot can be very soothing—try using a good old hot water bottle! A gentle massage might help. Other possibilities that may appeal to you are meditation and acupuncture.

Whatever means you use to control it, your pain will be more of a problem at some times than at others. It will probably seem much worse when you are bored, lonely, depressed, anxious, frightened, physically tired or lying awake at night (the worst). On the other hand, your pain is likely to seem less of a problem when you are in comfortable surroundings, have pleasant company, are keeping your mind occupied, sleeping well at night and at peace with yourself and your situation.

So, think about what *you* can do to take your mind off your pain and to reduce your feelings of fear and anxiety. Try to express and explore your feelings with family and friends and see if you can come to accept the aspects of your situation that you cannot change. Try to deal with your fear of the future by confronting it rather than by letting your imagination run riot. Fear feeds on the unknown. So ask a doctor, nurse, social worker or someone else you can trust about what is likely to happen to you. Ask them directly about any particular bogey you have—is it really likely to happen, and what could be done about it if it does? I am sure that if you can do this you will feel more at ease and your pain will be less of a problem for you.

If your pain proves really difficult to control, in spite of following the approaches I have recommended, think about what you are gaining from it. No, that's not a misprint, I do mean *gaining*. Are you frightened of being discharged from hospital? Does the fact that you still have pain mean you can stay there, where you feel safer? Does your pain mean that you are less likely to be left on your own? If something like this is happening for you, there may be other, much less unpleasant ways of getting what you need. Perhaps you could tell friends, family, nurses, social worker, chaplain or someone else you trust just what it is you need. Perhaps you could try to work out what it is about hospital that makes it feel safer and then see what you could do to make home feel safer. Perhaps you could ask to have someone to keep you company just because you're lonely and frightened, accepting that you don't need to have pain to ask for this. Basically, try to ask for what you need directly instead of through your pain. You may be surprised at the results.

Obstacles To Pain Relief

Let's now stop assuming that you have plentiful supplies of any painkiller and get onto the most common obstacle to good pain relief. As I have already indicated, the usual reason for people suffering from poorly controlled cancer pain is that their doctor fails to prescribe enough of a strong enough painkiller. Because all strong painkillers are available only on prescription, you are completely dependent on your doctor(s) to supply them. If you are in hospital, you are dependent both on the doctors and on the nurses for access to painkillers.

What can you do if you are denied access to enough painkillers to give you continuing pain relief? First of all, I'll remind you that the usual reason for doctors and nurses limiting supplies of pain-killers is not cruelty or sadism, but sheer ignorance! So you may be able to overcome your problem by telling your doctors and nurses some of the things you have learned here. I'm sure I don't have to warn you to try to be diplomatic about this—we all know how some doctors hate to feel that their authority is being under-mined in any way!

There are some doctors who will not listen, who will act in a disinterested and impatient way if you try to discuss your pain control with them and who clearly give pain control a low priority. If you have a doctor like this, you would probably be better off changing doctors, as we discussed in the introduction to this chapter. Unfortunately, there is no type of doctor that I can guarantee will be good at pain control. I believe that the ones who are most likely to be well informed about painkillers are doctors who specialise in pain control, in terminal or palliative care, in radiotherapy or chemotherapy treatment. You can ask for a second opinion from one or more doctors from whichever of these categories is available and seems appropriate for you. I hope you strike it lucky first time!

Right, let's say you now have a doctor who is interested and concerned about your pain. What if this doctor agrees that you need a certain dose of a certain painkiller, say 20 milligrams of physeptone, but tries to send you away with a prescription for twenty tablets of 10 milligrams each and an appointment in two weeks time. However concerned this doctor appears, he or she is making it impossible for you to take your painkillers in an ideal way — regularly. He or she is forcing you to ration yourself, to take them only when your pain is really bad. Don't let them do this. Tell them you understand it is best to take the painkillers regularly. Ask how long they last if you haven't already checked it for yourself. Don't leave the doctor's surgery without prescriptions for enough tablets to take the required dose, *every* six hours in this case, until your next appointment (in our example, this means you would need 112 tablets), or get a repeat prescription. You may not, in fact, take all of those tablets, but at least you are free to decide what's best for you. If you don't have the tablets, you don't have the choice.

In Britain, some painkillers can be bought over the counter (for example aspirin or paracetamol). However, registered doctors can prescribe any quantity of prescription only drugs or controlled drugs that he or she feels appropriate.

If you are in hospital, you have to rely on nurses as well as doctors to get the painkiller you need. First, ask your doctor to write up your painkiller to be taken regularly (every three to six hours as is appropriate for the particular painkiller), not 'as required'. If it is written up 'as required' you will have to ask for every dose. Even once you persuade the nurse you *do* need it, you will have to wait while senior nurses and keys are found, so cupboards can be unlocked to get your painkiller out. You shouldn't have to go through this and you won't have to if you can persuade your doctor to say you must have the painkiller regularly.

Your doctor may want to write you up for two, three or more different painkillers. It is much better to stick to a strong-enough dose of one painkiller, taken regularly, often enough to keep the pain under control. Tell your doctor you prefer this.

Your doctor may want to give you injections. This is not necessary unless you are vomiting, can't swallow or are too drowsy to take your painkillers by mouth. You can get just as good an effect with tablets or syrup as injections, but not with the same dose. You need two to four times as much by mouth as by injection in order to finish up with the same amount in the bloodstream. Make sure your doctor allows for this if you are changing from injections to tablets or syrup.

You must take responsibility for telling your doctor just how well or how poorly your pain is being relieved. So many people say 'Not too bad' in response to a question about pain relief from their doctors and then both parties leave it at that. You're the only one who knows how it feels and you must tell your doctor about it if you want relief. You have every right to tell your doctor things like these and to expect some positive action on them: 'You have prescribed my painkiller every six hours, but it only lasts about four hours for me', or 'The pain keeps me awake at night' or 'I'm comfortable only if I lie completely still and I expect better pain relief than that'.

Your doctor may respond by saying that what has been prescribed 'should' be enough. Such a reply implies that the poor pain relief is somehow your fault. Don't let your doctor make you feel guilty because you are still in pain. If you *are* still in pain, it is because you are not getting enough of a strong enough painkiller often enough—simple as that. It is your doctor's responsibility and duty to correct that situation and if he or she does not do so you have every right to complain and ask for immediate referral to another doctor. The fault does *not* lie with you.

Some doctors will refuse to increase, or will even reduce your dose of painkiller if *they* decide it is making you too drowsy. They may do this even though your pain is not controlled. I believe that you have the right to have enough painkiller to control your pain, especially if your cancer cannot be cured and the cause of your pain cannot be corrected. *You* should decide whether you would prefer to be more alert and in more pain or drowsier and in less pain, even though the decision to be drowsier could mean that you don't live quite as long as you would have otherwise. Your wishes in this regard are more likely to be respected if you talk to trusted family members or friends and your doctors about them *before* the situation ever arises. You could even put them in writing if you want to be as sure as possible that your last days will be as *you* want.

Special Procedures For Pain Relief

Finally, I'll just mention a few specialised ways of dealing with pain which could be recommended for you. Pain confined to one part of the body can sometimes be relieved by cutting or deadening the nerves that run between that part and the brain. With such methods you run a risk of also losing other feelings besides pain, like touch, and of losing the use of the muscles in that part of the body. For example, if the pain is in the pelvic area, you would risk losing feeling and strength in the leg(s) and control of the bowel and bladder.

If such an approach is recommended for you, ask exactly what is involved, how long you would have to spend in hospital, how likely it is to relieve your pain and for how long, and about the nature and likelihood of any side effects as well as how long they might last. The cost/benefit balance may well be worse than you can reach with painkillers. I certainly would not recommend these sorts of methods before you have tried using painkillers *as I have described*.

For extensive cancer pain, some doctors recommend an injection of morphine into the covering around the spinal cord through a small plastic tube which can be left in place (epidural injection). This can result in better pain relief for less side effects, but has some drawbacks such as the risk of infection, inconvenience, and the need for a practitioner who is experienced in placing the tube correctly.

Another specialised method for relieving cancer pain is destruction of the pituitary gland by inserting alcohol, ice cold probes or radioactive substances into it via the nose (see pages

294–95). The pain relief is *not* achieved through producing remission of the cancer. This method may therefore be recommended for any cancer pain, not just that due to a type of cancer which could be dependent on the hormone balance in the body. I would not agree to it for myself because I believe that it is too unreliable and temporary in its effects and that the side effects are too great for the benefits. However, you must weigh up the situation *for yourself* if it is recommended for you. I definitely wouldn't try it before trying painkillers *as I have described*.

GENERAL LACK OF ENERGY/FEELING TIRED ALL THE TIME

Having cancer is a very tiring business! I'd be very surprised if you had never experienced this symptom. The cancer itself can sap your energy, especially if it is extensive and/or you have lost some weight. Many complications of cancer cause general weakness and lack of energy—for example, anaemia; lungs, liver or kidneys that don't work properly; and too much calcium or too little sodium or potassium in the blood. All forms of cancer treatment can be very tiring. Of course, nervous tension and worry about the future can make you feel very tired and disinterested in any of your normal activities, even ones that you are physically well enough for.

It is worth checking for those factors that can be treated amongst the ones I have mentioned above if you feel particularly tired and lacking in energy. For example, anaemia can be righted with a blood transfusion. The mineral disturbances mentioned can all be corrected if they are found. Perhaps your anti-cancer treatment can be modified—ask about cutting down doses for example. You should also consider stopping your anti-cancer treatment altogether. Weigh the costs you are now experiencing against the likely benefits—your decision may not be the same as when you first agreed to have the treatment. Then you were working on what you were told was likely, now you can reconsider in the light of what is actually happening to you.

Nervous tension may be playing some part in producing your

lack of energy, especially if you are refusing to acknowledge or express some of your real feelings. It is when you try to force natural feelings like anger, sadness or anxiety underground that they are likely to surface in the form of unpleasant symptoms like extreme tiredness. Don't force yourself to appear bright, cheerful and optimistic when you don't really feel like that at all. Talk about and express your feelings—let them out and share them with your loved ones. I am sure that you will *all* have more energy to deal with what is happening if you can do this.

Try not to burn up energy raging against things that cannot be changed. Use what energy you have positively, to make the most of your situation. If you can no longer manage activities that have been important for you, think about whether you can modify them in some way so that you *can* manage. Ask for help— obstinately insisting on being independent could mean that you will miss out on some things that you could have managed with a bit of help. Look for appealing alternatives that *are* within your capabilities. In short, try to make the most of the time and energy that you do have. It is actually quite likely that you will *gain* energy as a result!

NAUSEA AND VOMITING

Nausea is feeling sick in the stomach and we all know what vomiting is!

As with all symptoms, the first thing to do if you develop nausea is to find out the reason for it. Here are some of the many possibilities. Nausea can be directly due to your cancer itself— such as when it is in the stomach area or liver, blocking the bowel or kidneys or in the brain (this last usually causes headache as well). Nausea can be due to cancer treatment—radiation, chemotherapy or too little corticosteroid hormone in the system (see pages 289–90). Cancer can also cause nausea indirectly, for example, through release of too much calcium in the blood (see page 134). Anxiety can itself cause nausea and can also aggravate nausea of any cause. Of course, don't forget that your nausea could be nothing to do with your cancer. For example, it could be caused by something you have eaten, a virus, gastritis, a stomach ulcer, or even a hangover!

It is important to consider every possible explanation. For example, just because you are having chemotherapy, you should not jump to the conclusion that any nausea you have is due to it. Chemotherapy-caused nausea usually follows a similar pattern for each course of treatment. If your pattern changes drastically, another reason should be looked for.

Once the cause(s) for your nausea are found, it may be possible to remove or correct them. For example, if it is due to the cancer itself, some form of anti-cancer treatment would be a possible, but not necessarily the best, way to tackle it. If it is due to cancer in the brain, corticosteroids could relieve the nausea temporarily by reducing the pressure on the brain (see page 286). If it is due to a bowel blockage, surgical removal or bypass of the blockage may be possible. If it is due to radiotherapy or chemotherapy it may be possible to change the doses, or even stop the responsible treatment. If it is due to, or aggravated by, anxiety, talking about and dealing with some of your worries, learning relaxation techniques and taking sedatives are three approaches you could consider.

The nausea itself must be treated if the cause is not to be removed — either because this is impossible or because you decide that the likely cost of removing the cause would outweigh the likely benefit. I suggest you read pages 240–42 here. This section is basically about the treatment of nausea due to chemotherapy, but the same sorts of approaches can be followed for nausea due to other reasons. Remember, there are a number of different anti-nausea medications and it can be a matter of trial and error to find the one that suits you best. Chemical names of some good ones are prochlorperazine, metoclopramide, thiethylperazine maleate and chlorpromazine.

LOSS OF APPETITE/LOSS OF WEIGHT

These two often go hand-in-hand, so I have put them under the same heading. Loss of appetite, with or without some nausea and/or change in how things taste is quite common in people with cancer. Often these symptoms are due to treatment rather than to the cancer itself, because both chemotherapy and radiotherapy can produce loss of appetite and weight. Of course, cancer itself can also cause loss of appetite and weight, especially when it is in the stomach area, liver or pancreas. However, it by no means *always* does so—loss of weight is *not* something that happens to everybody with extensive cancer. Some people never lose weight—not even in the final stages.

If your appetite is poor and/or some things now taste unpleasant, try to work out what tastes do appeal to you now and plan your diet accordingly. Don't force yourself to eat certain foods that you now find unpleasant just because you believe they are 'good for you'. Look for a more appealing alternative—for example, if you find meat distasteful, you may be able to get the protein you need from nuts, seeds, beans, dairy products and eggs.

If possible, eat small snacks of something appetising and nutritious often, rather than trying to push down three big meals each day. For example, you could try a cup of soup or a milk drink with a piece of cake instead of just a cup of tea or coffee between meals. Ask for a referral to a dietician if you want help and advice about making your restricted diet more nutritious and appetising. I suggest you also take multivitamin and mineral supplements to make sure that you don't miss out on any essentials. Small doses of corticosteroid drugs such as prednisolone can stimulate the appetite and make you feel generally more energetic. The dose needed to do this is usually so small that it is unlikely to cause any troublesome side effects. You could read about corticosteroids on pages 286–90 and ask your doctor about this if your appetite is very poor.

Some of you will be reading this section because you have the job of preparing meals for someone with cancer who has a poor and finicky appetite. Try to remember that if your friend or family member is losing weight, it is *not* your fault, nor is it their's. Your loved one may continue to lose weight in spite of your combined best efforts. If they do this, try not to take it personally. Their weight loss doesn't mean that you are not caring for them properly, nor does it mean that they are not grateful for your efforts and eating as much as they comfortably can of what you prepare. It is no more possible to stop some people with cancer from losing weight than it is possible to stop some people with cancer from dying of it.

So try to aim for what is possible. If you refuse to settle for anything less than stopping a person who has extensive cancer or is having very intensive chemotherapy from losing weight, you are likely to succeed only in making both of your lives miserable. Both of you have enough to deal with without getting into battles over food. Why not simply aim for pleasant meal times, free of nagging or feelings of guilt? Perhaps there are even times when both of you would benefit more from a chat and a cuddle than more food!

CONSTIPATION

You are constipated if your motions are hard and you have difficulty opening your bowels. It doesn't really matter if you don't open your bowels very often, as long as your motions are soft and easy to pass when you do.

I'm sure you know some of the simple things that can cause constipation—not eating enough (especially not enough fibre), not drinking enough fluids, and lack of exercise. Certain drugs can make the bowel work sluggishly, including most painkillers, the chemotherapy drugs vinblastine and vincristine and some antacids. The barium that is given by mouth for X-rays of the stomach and intestines or in enema form for X-rays of the lower bowel is also very constipating. Constipation is one of the symptoms caused by excessive calcium in the blood (see page 134).

Another possible cause for constipation is damage to the nerves which supply the muscle in the wall of the bowel. This can happen if you have a cancer growth pressing on the spinal cord or on the nerves as they pass through the pelvis. With constipation due to nerve damage, you may not be able to tell when you need to open your bowels. This is because the nerves which carry this message are often damaged along with the ones which supply the bowel muscle.

Constipation can also be caused by cancer directly, through partial or complete blockage of the bowel. Constipation due to blockage is often accompanied by pain and sometimes by passage of blood and/or small amounts of slimy fluid through the back passage. If the blockage is right down near the rectum you may feel as though you want to open your bowels all the time. This is because a growth inside the rectum or pressing on it can feel just like a motion always waiting there. I think it is easier to cope with this unpleasant symptom if you understand what is causing it. Of course, if you have hard motions in the rectum which you cannot pass without help, you can get exactly the same symptoms—a feeling as though you want to go all the time, but when you do, you pass only *small* amounts of slimy fluid. These symptoms are sometimes mistaken for diarrhoea, which can be disastrous— obviously treating it as diarrhoea can make it much worse! This mistake should never be made because it is very easy for a doctor or nurse to tell one from the other simply by checking inside your rectum with a gloved finger.

As with all symptoms, it is quite common for more than one factor to play a part in producing constipation. Once the cause(s) have been found, consider tackling them directly. It may be possible to treat a blockage by surgery, radiation or chemotherapy. However, the cost of doing so may outweigh the benefit if, for example, the treatment is unpleasant and has only a small chance of shrinking the growth enough to relieve the symptoms. If you either can't or don't want to get rid of the cause of your con- stipation—for example, because it is due to painkillers which you want to keep taking—you will have to tackle the symptom itself. Prevention is better than cure here. Don't wait until you are really badly constipated before doing something about it.

I suggest for a start you consider taking some form of laxative regularly. Laxatives work by softening the motion and/or stimulating the bowel muscle—good examples include liquid paraffin, phenolphthalein, dioctyl sodium sulphosuccinate, danthron, lactulose, and senna. If you normally take laxatives anyway, you will need much bigger doses now than someone who is not used to taking them. Other ways of helping the bowels to keep moving are by taking a high-fibre diet (but *not* if you have a blockage of the bowel), drinking plenty of fluids and exercising as much as is possible and comfortable.

If these measures don't keep your bowels moving easily, you may also need to use suppositories or enemas, with the help of a nurse. By the way, most nurses know much more about treating constipation than most doctors. I suggest that you ask a nurse for help if you have this symptom. This should be easy if you are in hospital. If you are at home, just ask your doctor to arrange for a nurse to visit you there.

DIARRHOEA

Diarrhoea means passing loose motions often and usually with urgency—in other words, you can't wait long once you get the urge to open your bowels.

Possible causes include infections, radiation treatment to the bowel, and some drugs—antibiotics, chemotherapy drugs, or overuse of laxatives. Diarrhoea can also be due to what we call malabsorption—here the bowel can't absorb certain substances into the blood from inside it. The diarrhoea of malabsorption often consists of large, pale, soft motions which contain a lot of fat. This makes them float and therefore hard to flush away. Causes of malabsorption include diseases (including cancer) of the liver, pancreas or small bowel, blockage of the tubes running from the liver or pancreas into the bowel and surgical removal of parts of the small bowel. Nervous tension can also cause diarrhoea, or aggravate it, whatever its original cause.

If your diarrhoea is due to infection, this should be treated. If it is due to radiation, your course of treatment could be adjusted—talk to your doctor about this. If your diarrhoea is due to chemotherapy drugs, you could consider reducing the dose or even cutting out the responsible drug altogether.

When diarrhoea starts during or soon after a course of antibiotics, it usually means that the antibiotics have killed all the useful bacteria which are normally in our bowel. When this happens, other harmful bacteria can take over. Stopping the responsible antibiotics and eating yoghurt (a source of useful bacteria) may be enough to get the bowel back to normal.

Diarrhoea due to malabsorption can often be corrected by a special diet and medications to help the bowel break down and absorb fats. If the malabsorption is due to blockage of the tubes running from the liver or pancreas to the bowel, it may be possible to correct this surgically. Just because it is possible does not necessarily mean it is best. Check the likely costs and benefits carefully.

Whether or not the cause of your diarrhoea is being tackled, you should take something to control it in the meantime. Anti-diarrhoea drugs work by slowing down the bowel muscle and/or making the motions more solid. Chemical names of some good ones include kaolin, pectin, codeine phosphate, aluminium hydroxide, loperamide hydrochloride and diphenoxylate hydro-chloride. It should be possible to improve diarrhoea greatly within less than a day with these drugs. If anti-diarrhoea treatment is not offered to you while the cause of your diarrhoea is being looked for or treated, ask for it.

It is important to make sure that you don't get dehydrated while you have diarrhoea. If it is severe or accompanied by nausea and vomiting, you might need intravenous fluids until it is brought under control.

If you have malabsorption, you could become deficient in certain vitamins (such as vitamins A, D and K) and minerals (such as calcium). Make sure your doctor checks these. You may need to take extra of some things, either by mouth or in injection form.

INABILITY TO PASS URINE
(Urinary Retention)

Inability to pass urine can be due to weakness of the bladder muscle or blockage of the passage running from the bladder to the outside. Weakness of the bladder muscle can arise from damage to or pressure on the nerves of the bladder—the trouble spot could be in the spinal cord or the pelvis. Such nerve damage usually causes loss of feeling in the bladder as well, so that you can't tell when it is full. You may also become unable to empty your bladder properly as a result of certain drugs such as the chemotherapy drug vinblastine, some anti-depressants and some drugs which are used to control diarrhoea or urinary incontinence (inability to hold the urine).

Cancer of the cervix or prostate can block the urinary passage. So can non-cancerous enlargement of the prostate gland. If you are unable to pass any urine at all naturally, it can be released either by passing a soft plastic tube (catheter) up through the urinary passage from the outside or by inserting a small tube through the skin of the lower part of your abdomen. Either of these can be comfortably done with the help of some local anaesthetic. The catheter may only be needed temporarily while the cause of the problem is tackled. If the cause cannot be corrected, or you decide that the cost of doing so would be greater than the benefit, you might have to keep a catheter permanently in place. This carries a risk of infection, but could still be the best alternative for you.

There are medications which can stimulate the bladder muscle to work better, for example, bethanechol chloride. With or without their help, you may be able to train yourself to empty a partially paralysed bladder naturally, so ask about this if the idea appeals to you.

PASSING URINE OFTEN

If you need to pass urine often, but pass only *small* amounts each time, and especially if it also stings or burns to pass it, the lining of your bladder is probably inflamed (cystitis). Possible reasons include infection, radiation to the pelvic area and the chemotherapy drug cyclophosphamide (see pages 257–59).

If you need to pass urine often in *large* amounts, you are producing too much urine. Possible causes include kidney failure, sugar diabetes (perhaps due to corticosteroids), diabetes insipides and too much calcium in the blood. Diabetes insipides is a condition where you pass large amounts of very weak urine. It can follow attempts to destroy the pituitary gland—see page 295.

Your doctor should quickly be able to find out why you are passing urine too often by testing your urine and blood.

I'll just explain a bit more here about one of the possible causes. Too much calcium in the blood is a complication of cancer which we have not discussed in detail so far. If this is the reason for you passing a lot of urine often, you are likely to have other symptoms as well—nausea, unusual thirst, a metallic taste in the mouth, constipation, muscle weakness, drowsiness and confusion. Too much calcium in the blood usually means that your cancer has spread to the bones, especially if your cancer started in the breast. However, the reverse is not true—in general, cancer does not usually cause excessive release of calcium when it spreads to the bones. Some particular types of cancer can also cause high calcium levels in the blood without spreading at all, but this is unusual. The ones that can do it include squamous cancer of the lung and cancers of the kidney and ovary.

Too much calcium in the blood can sometimes be treated by getting the responsible cancer into remission. Of course this may either be impossible or so costly that you decide that it is not worth trying. The main alternative is to work on reducing the high calcium levels, either instead of attacking the responsible cancer, or while you are waiting for anti-cancer treatment to work. Some of the ways of reducing high calcium levels include flushing the calcium through the system with a lot of intravenous fluids, or by using mithramycin (see page 267), phosphate mixtures taken by mouth or corticosteroids (see pages 286–87).

LOSS OF CONTROL OF URINE AND/OR FAECES
(Incontinence, Fistulas and Stomas)

No one likes to lose the ability to control the passage of urine or faeces (develop incontinence). In our society, many people who develop these symptoms feel ashamed and embarrassed and may even want to keep it a secret. These feelings are understandable, but not appropriate. It is *not* your fault if you can't control your bowel or bladder. These symptoms deserve as much attention as any other and you should not feel ashamed to ask for it.

Incontinence falls into two quite different groups. Firstly, there is loss of control of urine or faeces coming through the normal passages. Secondly, there is loss of control of urine or faeces because it is coming away through a passage that doesn't normally exist. This may be a passage created by your cancer (a fistula) or an artificial opening made surgically (a stoma).

Let's talk first about incontinence where urine or faeces is coming through the normal passages. This can basically develop for three different reasons, one or more of which could be operating in your case. Firstly, when you can't tell when your bladder or bowel is full. Secondly, when you can't control the muscles that empty the bladder or bowel. Thirdly, when the lining of the bladder or bowel is so inflamed that the muscle responsible for emptying it goes into spasm which you cannot control (urge incontinence).

The first and second reasons tend to go together, because you usually lose both feeling and muscle control when the nerves to the bladder or bowel are damaged. The trouble spot could be in the pelvis or spinal cord. If it is in the spinal cord you are likely to have some loss of strength and feeling in the legs as well.

Incontinence due to nerve damage can take a special form called **overflow** incontinence. Here the bladder muscle is so weakened that to start with you can't pass urine at all (see pages 132–33). Then the bladder gets so full that small amounts of urine start to leak away, quite out of your control. A similar thing can happen with the bowels—they can get stretched with motions which you cannot pass. At that stage, small amounts of slimy fluid may start to come away, again, quite out of your control. This form of incontinence in the case of the bladder can be mistaken for cystitis and in the case of the bowel can be mistaken for diarrhoea. Such mistakes will not be made if a doctor or nurse examines you properly, including examining inside your rectum and your vagina with a gloved finger. In fact, this form of examination is necessary to work out the reason for every form of incontinence.

If the pelvic muscles (rather than the muscle of the bladder itself) are weakened, you can get what we call stress incontinence. Here small amounts of urine come away when you sneeze, cough or laugh. This is much more common in women, whose pelvic muscles can be weakened by difficult childbirths or pelvic surgery. Oestrogen treatment (see pages 282–84) can cause or aggravate this symptom.

The third type of incontinence — **urge** incontinence — is when you know you need to go, but you can't get there quickly enough. This symptom is the case of the bladder often means cystitis — perhaps due to injection, bladder radiation or cyclophosphamide (see pages 257–59). In the case of the bowels it can go with severe diarrhoea of any cause.

Now let's go on to incontinence where urine or faeces is coming away through a passage that doesn't normally exist. This can happen if you have a large cancer in the pelvic area, which grows through to open up an abnormal passage between the bowel or bladder and the skin or vagina (a fistula). If the opening of the fistula is through the skin of the abdominal wall or down below, this problem is easy to diagnose — it is quite obvious that the urine or faeces is coming through an opening that normally doesn't exist. If the opening is into the vagina the diagnosis is more difficult. It shoud be suspected whenever small amounts of urine or faeces are coming away almost continuously, *but* you still have normal feeling in the bladder or bowel as the case may be. You could also be passing some of your urine and faeces normally, with normal control. Ask your doctor to check for a fistula if you think that urine or faeces is coming away through your front passage.

It can be very difficult to work out ways of keeping clean and pleasant if you have a fistula. Sometimes the best solution is to have an operation to channel the urine or faeces into a bag through a specially made opening in the abdominal wall (a stoma). Such an opening for urine is called an ileal bladder or nephrostomy and for faeces is called a colostomy. It can be much easier to collect the urine or faeces cleanly and comfortably into a bag when it is coming through a carefully placed stoma than when it is coming through a fistula. An operation to make a stoma may also be recommended if your bowel or urinary passages are completely blocked.

If you have any type of incontinence, fistula or stoma, there is no need to struggle by yourself to keep things clean. There is a big range of specially designed pads, bags, pants, bedding, and other devices available. You need the help of someone who knows all about them in order to work out what is best for you. Don't hesitate to ask whether there are either specially trained nurses and/or associations for people with this type of problem in your area. If there are, go to them for advice on the best way to manage your problem. If there are not, ask for the help of nurses, physio-therapists or occupational therapists. They are likely to know much more about the practicalities than a doctor is. Don't worry about offending your doctor—you have a problem that deserves the attention of an expert and that expert is not your doctor.

Remember that your GP or district nurse can probably advise you on whatever home-help you are eligible for.

ABDOMINAL SWELLING
(Bloating)

Swelling of your abdomen means there is something extra there that is not normally present. This can be either fluid, gas, or large cancer growths.

If fluid is the cause of the swelling, it is usually lying within the peritoneal cavity. The peritoneum is a fine double membrane that lines our abdominal cavity. Fluid can form between the two layers of this membrane (the peritoneal cavity) for example, when cancer cells start growing on it. This fluid is called ascites. Ascites can also be caused by liver diseases—both cancer and some non-cancerous conditions.

Severe bloating due to wind can develop when the bowel is partly or completely blocked. Abdominal swelling can also be due to cancer itself—perhaps greatly enlarging your liver, spleen, or kidney(s).

If your swelling is due to fluid, the resulting discomfort, lack of appetite, nausea and indigestion can usually be quickly and simply relieved by draining the fluid away. This can be done under a local anaesthetic through a plastic tube inserted through the abdominal wall. Unfortunately, the relief will be temporary unless something is done to stop the fluid from forming again. Reducing your salt intake and taking tablets to help you pass urine (diuretics) may help. Treating the responsible cancer itself, say with chemotherapy, may be an attractive possibility if you have a type of cancer which has a good chance of responding favourably to chemotherapy.

Another means of preventing the fluid from building up again is to inject either a chemotherapy drug or a radioactive substance into the peritoneal cavity. This is likely to cause fever and pain over the next day or so. Although some cancer cells may be killed, this method acts mainly by sealing the peritoneal cavity, so that there is no space left between the two layers of the peritoneal membrane for the fluid to collect in. Unfortunately, the stuff that is injected doesn't usually spread right through the peritoneal cavity, so this method is rarely successful in completely stopping fluid from reforming.

Another alternative is just to have the fluid drained off whenever it builds up enough to cause you unpleasant symptoms. This can result in loss of a lot of fluid, protein and minerals, depending on the type of fluid you are forming. Ask your doctor if this is likely to cause a problem in your case and if so, what should be done to replace what you are losing.

BREATHLESSNESS

Feeling short of breath basically means that you are not getting enough oxygen into your blood. This could be because there is something wrong with the lung tissue itself—cancer in the lung, clots on the lung, pneumonia, radiation reaction, lung damage caused by bleomycin (see pages 255–56), or fluid building up in the lung because your heart is not working efficiently. Breathlessness can also be due to the lung being squashed by fluid building up outside it in what we call the pleural cavity (the membrane-lined space between the lung and the chest wall). Partial blockage of some of the bronchial tubes can also make you feel short of breath. The blockage could be caused by cancer pressing on them or spasm (as happens with asthma). Breathlessness can also be a symptom of anaemia. When you are anaemic, your blood does not carry as much oxygen as normal, so you automatically breathe faster to try to get more oxygen into the blood. And, of course, nervous tension can result in a feeling of breathlessness, or aggravate breathlessness of any other cause.

To find out which cause applies in your case your doctor should check for other symptoms. For example, if you are coughing yellow or green phlegm it is probably infection. If you are coughing blood, it could be cancer or blood clots on the lung. If you feel more short of breath when lying flat than when sitting or standing, your heart is probably not working properly. If you or your doctor can hear whistling sounds with your breathing, you probably have some partly blocked bronchial tubes.

Often your doctor will be able to tell the cause just by taking your history, examining you and arranging a chest X-ray, but sometimes other tests, such as a lung scan, may be advisable.

Once the cause is found, it may be possible to correct it. For example, pneumonia could be treated with antibiotics, clots on the lung with drugs to thin the blood (anticoagulants) and anaemia with a transfusion.

If your heart is the problem there are pills or injections which can make it work more efficiently and also ones to help you pass some of the fluid that has built up in the lungs out through the urine. Your doctor should also find out why it is not working properly—important possibilities to check in people with cancer include heart damage due to adriamycin (see pages 252–53) and fluid building up in the sac that surrounds the heart (the pericardial cavity). If the latter is the problem, your symptoms can be quickly improved by draining the fluid out through a needle or fine plastic tube put in through the chest wall under local anaesthetic. The needle does not go into the heart itself, just the fluid-filled sac around it. Fluid in the pleural cavity (outside the lungs) can also be drained in a similar way to produce a rapid improvement in your breathing.

If fluid has built up in either your pericardial or pleural spaces, cancer cells growing on their linings is the most likely reason, but other possible reasons include infection and bleeding. The fluid can be examined under the microscope to find out why it has formed. If it is due to cancer, ways of trying to stop it reforming are the same as for fluid in the abdominal cavity (ascites)— see page 138.

Breathing extra oxygen will make you feel easier, whatever the reason for your breathlessness. Ask about this if the reason for your breathlessness cannot be corrected, or if you feel that the cost of trying to correct it is too great for the likely benefit, or while you are waiting for treatment of the cause to work. It is quite feasible to have an oxygen cylinder at home and it also comes in small cylinders which can be fixed to a wheelchair or carried around fairly easily.

Feeling very breathless can be extremely frightening and stressful. You may find it very hard to relax or to sleep, even with oxygen. Having somebody sit with you may help. Taking a sedative is another possibility. In considering whether to take sedatives you should understand that they could make your breathing and coughing less efficient. This is a cost that you may well be prepared to accept, especially if your cancer cannot be cured and the reason for your breathlessness cannot be relieved. Some doctors take this choice out of their patient's hands, either by prescribing a sedative without telling them or by refusing to prescribe one even when the patient asks for it. The choice should be *yours*. Insist that your doctors prescribe nothing without your agreement. Tell them if you would prefer to be either more alert or more drowsy than you are. You have the right to choose, even if the choice to be more drowsy could mean that you don't live quite as long.

COUGH

Some of the things that can cause a dry cough are pressure on the windpipe or bronchial tubes, radiation reaction, bleomycin reaction (see pages 255–56) and fluid on the lungs (pleural fluid). A moist cough that produces yellowish or greenish phlegm is usually due to infection. A cough that produces blood could be due to cancer itself or to clots on the lung.

Treating the cause of your cough is one possibility to consider. What about if this is not possible, or you decide that its cost is too great or while you are waiting for the treatment of the cause to work?

If you have a lot of mucus, it is important to get rid of it and not to try to stop the cough. Inhaling steam, perhaps with menthol, camphor, eucalyptus etc added can help to moisten your air passages and make the phlegm easier to cough up. Make sure you keep drinking plenty of fluids as well. There are medicines, such as bromhexine HCl which are designed to make phlegm less sticky. Physiotherapy can also play an important part in helping you to get the phlegm up.

There are medicines to help dry up phlegm. They can have the disadvantage of making it stickier so that it is harder to cough it up. They will also give you a dry mouth and nose. Chemical names of some of these are pseudoephedrine HCl, phenylephrine HCl, atropine sulphate and hyoscine hydrobromide. The first two make some people feel unpleasantly agitated and restless, so ask what is in your cough medicine and whether you can have a different one if you have this symptom.

If your cough is dry, it is safe to take medicines to try to stop it. Chemical names of some are pholcodine, codeine phosphate and dextromethorphan hydrobromide. These are closely related to pain-killers, in fact some of them are quite good painkillers as well.

They can cause similar side effects, especially constipation, nausea, and drowsiness. For the first of these it is best to take preventive steps as described on pages 130–31. The other two tend to wear off, so persevere for a few days before deciding that these medicines don't suit you.

Quite a lot of cough mixtures contain antihistamines, which are not of much help for a cough from any of the causes listed above. Antihistamines may make you either drowsy or overactive and restless. Ask whether one is in your cough medicine if you get these symptoms, and if so, ask to have a different cough mixture that does not contain an antihistamine.

HEADACHE

Things that are nothing to do with cancer such as nervous tension, migraines and sinus problems can of course cause headaches in people with cancer, just as they can in anyone. However, the cause we will discuss here is the one that is likely to worry you the most — cancer in the brain or cerebro-spinal fluid (the fluid that surrounds the brain and spinal cord — CSF for short).

Cancer in these places causes headaches by increasing the pressure on the brain. These headaches are often accompanied by nausea, vomiting, and blurred vision. They tend to be worst when you have been lying down for a while and better when you are up and about. Cancer in the brain is a likely reason for headaches that are accompanied by double vision, pins and needles or numbness down one side or weakness in one side. Cancer in the CSF may be accompanied by a stiff back and neck, pains shooting into the arms and legs, and pins and needles, numbness or weakness in any or all limbs.

If you have headaches your doctor should examine you, including looking into your eyes to see whether the pressure on the brain is high. This is not a foolproof test — the back of the eye can look perfectly normal when the pressure on the brain is raised. A brain scan or CT scan will probably be needed in order to be sure of the reason for your headaches. A lumbar puncture will also be necessary if cancer in the CSF is suspected (see pages 79–80).

There is no type of cancer that can be cured once it has spread to the brain or cerebro-spinal fluid. Radiation treatment and/or injection of certain chemotherapy drugs into the CSF (see pages 226–27) may bring about temporary improvement in symptoms through temporary control of the cancer but *not* a complete and permanent cure.

There are also ways of temporarily relieving the symptoms of high pressure on the brain which do not involve treating the responsible cancer. Treatment with corticosteroids (see page 286) can reduce the swelling *around* cancer in the brain and so reduce the pressure. Corticosteroids will often get rid of nausea, headache, pins and needles and weakness caused by cancer in the brain or CSF within twenty-four hours. Of course, the relief is never permanent, but it can last for some months. An alternative to corticosteroids is glycerol (glycerine). Ask to try it if corticosteroids are either not working or producing side effects which you are not prepared to put up with. It is an extremely sweet syrup which is best taken with something bitter like grapefruit juice. Some people have no side effects from glycerol while others get nausea which is so troublesome that it outweights the benefits. You will know after the first couple of doses whether this is going to be a problem for you.

CONVULSIONS (Fits, Seizures)

The possibility of having fits is a frightening one I know, but they are not as bad as they look. They are not painful, they usually last only a few minutes, and you are not likely to die while having one.

A fit happens when part or all of the brain becomes abnormally irritable. If it is only part of the brain, there may just be jerky movements of part of the body—say one arm or leg—without loss of consciousness. A generalised fit involves jerking movements of the whole body and loss of consciousness for a few minutes. There may be some warning immediately before the fit in the form of strange feelings—anxiety, flashing lights, unusual smells, noises in the head or some other unusual feeling. When people come to from a fit they usually feel rather strange and tired for some hours and just want to sleep. Some part of their body may be paralysed when they first come to but this usually goes back to normal over the next few hours.

Fits starting in otherwise normal children or young adults are usually due to epilepsy and do not usually mean there is any disease of the brain. However, fits starting in an adult with cancer usually mean one of the following. Either part of the brain is damaged, perhaps by cancer, a stroke, or injury, or there is some abnormality in the mineral balance or purity of the blood which is causing unusual irritability of the brain. For example, extremely low levels of sodium or calcium or excessive wastes in the blood (such as can happen when the kidneys or liver are very badly damaged) can cause fits.

If you have a fit, your doctor must take your history, examine you carefully and do blood tests and perhaps a brain scan in order to find out the reason. If the reason is an abnormality in the blood, correcting this will prevent more fits. If the disorder cannot be corrected or if the fits are due to cancer or some other disease of your brain, they can be prevented only by taking drugs called anti-convulsants. Chemical names of some good ones include phenytoin sodium, phenobarbitone and clonazepam. It is important to understand that if your fits are due to cancer in your brain, they will not stop simply as a result of lowering the pressure on the brain with corticosteroids or glycerol. You will need anti-convulsants as well. By the way, many people with cancer in the brain never have fits, so don't expect this will necessarily happen if you have cancer in your brain.

Here are a few do's and don'ts for friends or relatives of someone who has fits. First of all, try not to panic. As I've said, fits usually last only a few minutes and your friend or relative is not likely to die while having one. When a fit starts, remove any hard or otherwise dangerous objects from nearby. Don't hold the person in an attempt to stop the jerking movements. Don't try to force his or her mouth open with a hard object — this is likely to do more damage than the biting of the tongue you are trying to prevent. Loosen any tight clothing, especially around the neck and chest. Once you can do this without causing injury (usually once the jerky movements have stopped), turn your friend or relative onto one or another side with his or her face pointing slightly downwards, until he or she comes to. This position ensures that the person's tongue is not blocking the air passages and that any fluid in his or her throat and mouth drains out. I suggest you ask a nurse to show you how to place someone in this position, so that you feel confident about it. Don't offer anything to eat or drink until your friend or relative has come to completely. Keep him or her nice and warm and respect his or her need to have a good sleep afterwards. That's not so difficult is it? I hope you don't feel quite so nervous about it now that you have some idea of what to do.

AGITATION AND RESTLESSNESS

Extreme agitation and restlessness are not always due to nervous tension. These symptoms can be caused by certain drugs—anti-nausea drugs, some sedatives, some cough mixtures and medicines designed to dry up phlegm, and corticosteroids. So, if you get these symptoms, especially if they start quite suddenly, ask your doctor to check through your medicines for any that could be causing it. The culprit will usually be one you have just started taking.

PRESSURE SORES (Bed Sores)

It is very important for you to read this section carefully if you can't move around freely and easily, *whether or not* you are confined to bed. You don't have to be in bed to get bed sores, which is why I prefer the name of pressure sores.

Pressure sores are nearly always preventable—you are not likely to get any if you, and the people caring for you, understand what causes them and how to prevent them. You are in danger of developing pressure sores whenever you stay in the same position for many hours at a time, especially if you have lost a lot of weight. This is because when weight is taken by any part of you where there is very little tissue between the skin and the bone, the circulation to that part may be cut off. It's not only your backside that is in danger. Pressure sores can develop on hips, knees, ankles, elbows, and even the back of the head—anywhere where there is bone very close to the skin.

They will not develop if you change your position often, keep dry, put some sort of padding over these danger points and get someone to massage them briskly, often. All of that is easier said than done. It is not much fun to change your position often if you are in pain and especially if there is only one position that is really comfortable for you. It is hard to change position often if you are partly paralysed or so weak that you can't do it without help. It is hard to keep dry if you are incontinent. It can be fiddly to try to arrange padding over your danger points. You might feel reluctant to ask busy nurses, friends, or relatives to spend time helping you to change position and rubbing any sore areas to help restore a brisk circulation. However, it *is* worth taking all of this seriously. Things are likely to be even more difficult for you if you do develop a pressure sore, because then you won't be able to sit or lie in the position that produced your sore at all!

This is another area where nurses, physiotherapists and occupational therapists are likely to be of very much more practical help than doctors. If you actually already have developed, or do develop, a pressure sore, you will certainly need this help to get it healed. But don't leave it until then to ask for advice. If you can't move around freely and easily, ask these people for help with choosing and getting into good positions, with ways to keep dry, with easy to manage ways of padding your danger points and with ideas of what to rub on any sore spots. You are unlikely to develop any pressure sores if you follow their advice.

Chapter 7

SURGERY

EXERCISING YOUR RIGHT TO MAKE YOUR OWN DECISIONS ABOUT SURGERY

For many types of cancer, complete surgical removal of the primary tumour is the only treatment that is ever capable of producing a complete and permanent cure. Surgery cures more cancers than does any other form of treatment. Surgery is also recommended to cancer patients for other reasons: to make a diagnosis, to relieve or prevent symptoms and to reconstruct parts of the body. We will look at each of these in turn later in this chapter.

There is one basic problem with surgical treatment which does not apply with other types of treatment. Surgery is done while you are unconscious and therefore incapable of making any decisions.

If something unexpected is found during an operation on you, decisions about the best immediate course of action will be taken out of your hands. They will be made on your behalf by the surgeon. Most surgeons take it for granted that they should be making all the decisions, so they have no strong reasons for trying to prevent this situation from arising. There is only one way to make sure that *you* make the decisions about what operation will be done. You must make sure that you know, as completely and accurately as possible, *before your operation* what will be found when you are opened up, and what can be done to deal with this situation. The more careful and thorough your pre-operative assessment is, the greater the possibility of the exact operation that you agree to being performed.

This is very important—so important that I will be repeating it, with examples, a number of times during this chapter.

Balancing Cost Against Benefit

As with any treatment, you need to weigh the likely 'benefit' against the likely 'cost'. These are some of the questions to which you will need answers:

- What is the aim of the surgery?
- What is the chance of achieving that aim?
- Would there be a better chance of achieving that aim if I had other forms of treatment as well as, or instead of, the surgery?
- How would I look afterwards? (You can ask to see photos of patients who have had the proposed operation.)
- What would be removed or damaged?
- How would my body function without these parts?
- Can other parts of my body take over the function of the removed or damaged parts?
- Is there some artificial means of doing this? If so, what exactly would it involve for me?
- What is the risk of dying during or soon after the operation?
- What complications are likely?
- Can they be treated?
- Would they be temporary or permanent?
- How long would I be in hospital?
- How long, if ever, before I would return to normal?

You will get the most accurate answers to these questions from surgeons who have a lot of experience with the particular operation under consideration. These surgeons are also most likely to 'deliver the goods', that is, to carry out the proposed operation skilfully and to actually achieve the promised results. Ask your surgeon how many of these particular operations he or she has done, *whether or not* you suspect lack of experience because you are getting vague or evasive answers to your questions. Ask if there are surgeons in your area who specialise in this type of operation. If there are, ask for a referral to them. Don't settle for an inexperienced surgeon because you don't wish to give offence. Your health and comfort are more important than that.

Remember, there are always alternatives. Ask about these if they are not volunteered. What other forms of treatments are possible, including those whose aims are not the same as the proposed surgery? What is the likely benefit and likely cost of each? Don't forget there is *always* the possibility of having no anti-cancer treatment at all. This possibility will rarely be mentioned, so you will probably have to ask directly. Try to find out what is likely to happen if you have no actual anti-cancer treatment.

Some Facts About Cancer Surgery

You may be frightened of having any operation at all for cancer because you have heard that 'letting the air in' makes the cancer grow and spread much more quickly. What facts support this belief? How heavily should it weigh when you are considering the possible costs of a proposed operation?

It is true that some people die of cancer very soon after having an operation for it. If you look into it you will find that most of these patients have had operations which consisted simply of opening them up, having a look and closing them up again. In other words, most of these patients already had extensive cancer *before* their operation, so extensive that no useful procedure was possible. Rather than asking 'Did the operation aggravate their cancer?', I think questions such as these are more important: 'What was the purpose of operating at all?' 'What possible benefit was expected?' 'Couldn't they have found out *before* operating that it would not be possible to do anything useful?'

'Open and shut' operations should hardly ever happen. They can usually be avoided by careful assessment of patients. The diagnosis and probable extent of disease should be established by tests before any operation is planned. A properly-planned procedure is rarely made impossible by finding something unexpected when the patient is operated on. Emergency operations are one exception to this, as we will see later in this chapter.

This is not to say that having an operation cannot possibly

result in some patients dying of cancer a bit sooner than they would have otherwise. For example, it is known that anaesthetics and stress depress the function of the immune system. Experiments on animals with extensive cancer have shown that those that have a 'look and see' operation do die, on average, a little earlier than animals which do not. Notice that I said animals having a 'look and see' operation, *not* animals having an operation at which something is done to the cancer.

Try to keep these facts in perspective. If your cancer is apparently localised, surgery probably offers you the best, and maybe the only, chance of cure. If it is extensive, surgery could be the best way of controlling or preventing very unpleasant symptoms. If you stand to gain a lot from surgery, the possible temporary effects of the stress and anaesthetic on your immune system would not be enough to outweigh the probable benefit. On the other hand, they could be if your planned operation has only a small chance of achieving some minor and temporary benefit.

Ensuring Full Evaluation Before Surgery

As with other treatments, so it is with surgery—no one can look into the future and tell you exactly what will happen to you as an individual. In the case of surgery, they can't even always tell you exactly what the operation will involve.

Let's start with an example. Say a person agreed to removal of part of the lower bowel, on the understanding that this would give him a good chance of being cured of bowel cancer altogether. At the operation, his surgeon finds something that was not known before the operation—the cancer has grown through the bowel wall and into the wall of the bladder. The cancer cannot be completely removed without removing part of the bladder as well. Even if this is done, the chance of cure is much smaller than was advised beforehand. This surgeon has two choices. He or she can take the decision away from the patient by going ahead immediately with whatever operation seems best. This is what most surgeons do. Or the surgeon could simply sew the patient up again and discuss the new situation with him when he wakes up. Clearly this wouldn't be good for the sick person, who would then have to consider having another operation within a very short time. It also wouldn't be good for the surgeon. The average surgeon is much too concerned with maintaining his or her power and authority over the patient to even consider such a course of action. Doing this would mean admitting lack of care in planning the operation. More importantly, it would also mean acknowledging that the person having the operation was indeed the best person to make the decision.

Steps can be taken to prevent such a situation from arising in the first place. Your surgeon can greatly reduce the chance of finding something unexpected during an operation by checking you carefully beforehand. This means getting a detailed history of your symptoms, examining you carefully, and arranging, with your agreement, whatever tests are necessary to provide a complete picture. In the example I have described, there would probably have been bladder symptoms such as burning, or passing urine more frequently, and/or in smaller amounts than normal. There may have been obvious blood passed or if not, traces of blood would probably have been found in the urine by testing. Special contrast X-rays or endoscopic examination of the bladder (cystoscopy) could have confirmed bladder involvement by the cancer. If the true situation had been established *before* operating, this person could have had control over the treatment decision, and the surgeon would not have been placed in a dilemma.

Here is how to be as sure as possible that your surgeon will be able to carry out the operation you have agreed to. When your surgeon recommends a certain operation, ask how sure he or she is that this operation will be possible. For example, if the aim of the operation is complete removal and possible cure, ask whether the diagnosis of cancer is definite and the exact type known. Ask whether the cancer has already spread into nearby organs. Have the appropriate tests been done to check this? How does your type of cancer usually spread? How sure are they that it as not already spread to nearby lymph glands or through the bloodstream? How can the likely sites for secondary growths be checked? These questions apply in the case of potentially curative surgery. Later in this chapter I will give you some idea of what should be known before attempting surgery that has various other aims.

Anticipating And Dealing With The Unexpected

Even when all possible care has been taken, something unexpected may still be found during an operation. This happens especially with emergency operations, when there is not enough time to completely evaluate the situation before operating. However, it can happen with any operation. This means that you need another safeguard. You need to know what *might* still be found that would make the proposed operation inadvisable or impossible. Ask directly. You need to know how your surgeon would want to deal with each possible situation. Again, ask directly. You have the right to *set limits* on what you will permit. For example, you may not be prepared to have your breast removed (mastectomy) or to have your bowel ending in an opening on the abdominal wall (colostomy) or to have both ovaries or both testicles removed. Before making a final decision, try to find out what would be likely to happen if you refuse a certain procedure. In other words, try to make a really informed decision when setting your limits. Horrified as you may be at the idea of a colostomy or mastectomy, it is possible that the consequences of *not* having these procedures could be worse.

Consent To Surgery—Protecting Your Rights

If you decide there is a certain procedure you will not allow under any circumstances, make sure that you tell your surgeon so very clearly, both orally and in writing. Read the consent form that you are asked to sign prior to your operation very carefully. On the form you are expected to agree not only to the operation, but also to further alternative operative measures which, in the opinion of the surgeon performing the operation may be found to be necessary during the course of the operation. *Unless you agree, do not sign this form as it stands—write in the procedure that you will not permit. Sign your addition* in the presence of a witness, as well as signing at the bottom of the form.

Alternatively, if you wish to ensure that only the operation you have agreed to and *nothing* else is done, you would also have to make this very clear to your surgeon beforehand. Tell him or her directly. In addition, cross out the disclaimer on your written consent form, write 'only' next to the name of the operation, and sign this as well as signing at the bottom of the form. In this way you will be giving consent only to the operation that is named on the form. If a technical name is written on the form, ask for it to be explained fully. You could even cross it out and write a description in your own words of the operation you *are* agreeing to if you want to be quite sure that your wishes are clearly understood.

So far, we have discussed putting limits on what your surgeon can do in an unexpected situation. The same considerations apply if your surgeon recommends, as the treatment of choice, a procedure that you are not prepared to undergo. You, as a responsible adult, have the right to refuse any form of treatment that you don't want, even if such refusal could mean that your life is likely to be shortened. No one has the right to override your refusal to any procedure, even when it could temporarily extend your life.

Of course, this, like so many things, is easier said than done! Your surgeon may be hurried, impatient and irritable with you. Your surgeon may tell you that he or she simply can't understand how anyone could make such a stupid decision. Your surgeon may appear to be insulted, disappointed or hurt because you are rejecting his or her advice. Don't be deterred by such reactions. You *do* know that there are limits to what you are prepared to sacrifice in order to live a bit longer. You probably know that even dying could be a better alternative for you than some types of drastic treatment. Trust what you know about yourself. You *do* know what's best for *you*.

DIAGNOSTIC SURGERY

How And Why Diagnosis Should Be Separated From Treatment

You will remember that a definite diagnosis of cancer cannot be made without examining cells from the suspicious area under the microscope. I explained in Chapter 3 how the necessary specimens can be obtained.

An actual operation is not usually necessary to make the diagnosis of cancer. Making a diagnosis and having treatment are two quite separate things. Most often the diagnosis can, and should, be definitely proved *before* any treatment, including surgical treatment, is planned. This is because it is not possible to decide on the best possible treatment until the diagnosis of cancer is confirmed and the particular type known.

What can happen if the diagnosis is not established before operating? Say a patient has a shadow on their chest X-ray which looks very like cancer. One way of definitely finding out would be to remove all or part of the lung—combining diagnosis and treatment in one procedure. Afterwards, when the removed lung is examined under the microscope it might indeed be found to contain primary lung cancer. However, it is also possible that it could contain a secondary cancer deposit from some other part of the body or even some type of infection or inflammatory reaction. Although removal of the lung certainly allows a definite diagnosis to be made, we know that there are far less drastic ways of making a diagnosis! In addition, removal of the lung is not even the best form of treatment for all types of primary lung cancer. It is certainly not the best form of treatment for any of the other conditions that might have been found.

Many surgeons recommend that the two steps are carried out separately but *under the same anaesthetic*. For example, patients with suspected breast cancer are often asked to agree to be put to sleep, following which the surgeon takes a sample of the suspicious area. This is rapidly examined under the microscope by a process called frozen section. Once the diagnosis is made, the surgeon immediately proceeds to carry out whatever operation he or she considers best.

It is neither necessary nor best *for you* to do things this way. In the case of breast lumps, the diagnosis can be made pre-operatively by a needle biopsy. With most types of cancer it is possible to make the diagnosis and carry out any surgical treatment in two completely separate steps. This has two major advantages. Firstly, it allows time for the biopsy to be fully processed and examined. The rapid frozen section method used during operations is fairly accurate. However, it is not as reliable as the usual process, which takes several days. The pathologist can *usually* tell whether or not it is cancer but it less likely to tell the exact type of cancer on frozen section. The type of cancer is often very important in determining the best type of treatment. The other big advantage of making the diagnosis separately is that this gives you the opportunity to decide on the best possible treatment knowing all the important facts.

If diagnosis and treatment are combined in the one operation, you cannot be in control of the treatment decision. You must agree to the surgeon carrying out whatever operation seems best once the diagnosis is made. You are put to sleep not knowing what operation will be done. Whether or not your surgeon attempts to discuss all the various possibilities with you beforehand, this is not a good option for you. It means you are likely to be unnecessarily disturbed and confused by having to consider a whole lot of different possibilities before your operation.

Why do surgeons recommend the frozen section type of procedure then? They recommend it because it is easier for them and because they take it for granted that *they* should decide what operation is best. Do all you can to ensure that the diagnosis is made *before* you agree to a treatment-type operation.

When Diagnosis Cannot Be Separated From Treatment

There are some cases when all efforts to make a pre-operative diagnosis are either unsuccessful or prevented by the urgency of the situation. Here is an example of the first type of situation. A person has had persistent abdominal pain and weight loss, for which no cause can be found on clinical examination and extensive tests. Cancer is suspected but cannot be proved. An exploratory operation may be recommended. In this case the person must either be prepared to have two major abdominal operations within a few days of each other, or agree to the surgeon immediately performing whatever operation seems best once the diagnosis is made. Fortunately, it is rarely so difficult to make a diagnosis. If such an exploratory operation is recommended to you I suggest that you ask for a second opinion before agreeing to it. Another doctor may be able to think of a way of making the diagnosis without operating.

The other type of situation where it is not always possible for you to be in control is the emergency one. Say a person suddenly develops severe abdominal pain, bloating, and vomiting and can't pass anything through the back passage. Clinical examination and X-rays show that the bowel is completely blocked and that it has burst, leaking air and bowel contents into the abdominal cavity. The underlying problem could be cancer, but it would be dangerous to spend time trying to make a definite diagnosis before operating. This is one situation where there is no real alternative to letting the surgeon combine the diagnosis and *initial* treatment in one procedure. It is only once the person is opened up and the cause of the problem discovered, that decisions can be made on how best to deal with it. This isn't so bad when you realise that emergency surgery is rarely more than the first step in the treatment of any cancer. Once the emergency situation has been dealt with, there should be plenty of time to get all the information you need to make a considered decision on the best follow-up treatment for the cancer itself.

Remember, any person, including one facing emergency surgery, still has a right to know beforehand what is likely to be found and how the surgeon will probably want to deal with it. Any person also has a right to set limits on what he or she will permit. We discussed this earlier in this chapter. For example, the emergency patient described above may not wish to have a colostomy (bowel emptying through an opening on the abdominal wall). He or she has the right to refuse a colostomy and also the right to know what could happen because of such a refusal. Refusal may not create a problem if the surgeon can relieve the obstruction by some other means, such as removing or bypassing the blocked section of bowel. However, if this is not possible, the person's refusal to have a colostomy could mean his or her death within a few days of the operation. Knowing this, he or she is *still* entitled to refuse a colostomy. No surgeon has the right to override an adult patient's refusal to agree to any procedure, even though that procedure could be temporarily life saving. You know what's best for you. You know what you can and can't handle. You may know that you would rather die than have some drastic temporarily life saving treatment. Hold on to what is right for you.

POTENTIALLY CURATIVE SURGERY

Here is a self-evident, but very important fact. Surgery can only cure you if all of your cancer is removed. What circumstances are necessary for complete removal to be possible? The primary cancer must be confined to a part of the body that can safely be partly or completely removed. The primary cancer must not have extended directly into surrounding organs that cannot be removed. If it has spread through the lymph system, it must be possible to remove, preferably all in one piece, the primary cancer and the involved nodes. The cancer must not have spread through the blood system at all. How can we be as sure as possible, before operating, whether or not complete removal is feasible? First, we will look only at *feasibility*. Later we will consider *desirability*, that is, whether the cost/benefit balance is in favour of the surgery.

What Cancers Can Be Cured By Surgery?

First of all, there are some types of cancer for which complete surgical removal is never feasible. Cancers which start in many different parts of the body at the same time can never be cured surgically. Examples include leukaemias and myeloma (cancers of the bone marrow) and most lymphomas (cancers of the lymph nodes). The other group of cancers which cannot be cured surgically are those starting in a part of the body which is essential to life and the function of which cannot be naturally or artificially replaced. Examples include cancers of most parts of the brain, spinal cord, heart, and cancers which extensively involve the liver.

Then there are some types of cancer which can rarely be cured by surgery on its own because they almost always release cells into the bloodstream very early, before the primary cancer is big enough to be detected. Examples include some primary bone cancers (Ewing's sarcoma, osteogenic sarcoma), small cell anaplastic (oat cell) cancer of the lung, cancer of muscle (rhabdomyosarcoma), a type of kidney cancer (Wilm's tumour) and others. With these types of cancer you will make the best decisions if you simply take it for granted that tiny blood-borne seedlings *are* present, even when no actual secondary growths can be detected. Obviously these types of cancer are rarely cured simply by removal of the primary growth. Usually the best chance of cure is provided by chemotherapy combined with either surgery and/or radiotheraphy treatment.

We have some organs which can be partly or completely removed, even though they have functions which *are* essential to life. Removal is possible because there are ways of naturally or artificially restoring the functions of these organs. Sometimes this is possible because the organs have a lot of reserve. For example, if ninety per cent of your liver is removed, the other 10 per cent, provided it is normal, can do everything that the whole liver used to do. If certain parts of your stomach or intestines are removed, digestion and elimination of waste products can still be good enough to keep you at your normal weight. The remaining intestine may need some help in the form of a special diet or medications that assist digestion of certain foods. Some hormone glands, such as the thyroid gland, can be completely removed because the hormones it normally produces can be taken in tablet form.

Sometimes the part to be removed can be reconstructed. For example, part of the oesophagus (gullet) can be removed and replaced with a piece of intestine. The bladder can be removed and replaced by an artificial one made of a piece of intestine, emptying through an opening in the abdominal wall into a bag (an ileal bladder). The rectum and anus can be removed and the remaining bowel made to empty into a bag through an opening in the abdominal wall (a colostomy).

Luckily we have two of some of the organs whose functions are essential to life—for example, kidneys, lungs and adrenal glands. One healthy kidney, lung or adrenal gland can keep our bodies functioning quite normally.

There are many organs and parts of the body which are not essential to life. Although, of course, their loss results in varying degrees of mutilation, inconvenience and psychological distress, we *can* live without things like an arm, a leg, an eye, a tongue, a larynx (voice-box), a breast, an ovary, a testicle or a uterus (womb).

Checking Extent Of Cancer Before Attempting Potentially Curative Surgery

Say you do have a cancer which is in a part of the body that can be safely removed. How can you be as sure as possible, before the operation, that complete removal of the cancer is feasible? Firstly, you should understand that if only the visible cancer growth is removed, without a margin of apparently normal tissue, it is most unlikely that you will be cured. This is because of the ability of cancer cells to grow into the surrounding tissues. They do this in small columns or clumps which are much too tiny to be seen other than through a microscope. Before the operation, then, it is important to know just where the borders of your primary cancer growth appear to be. Your surgeon will then know whether or not it will be possible to remove an adequate margin of the apparently normal tissues surrounding it. Your doctor should check the apparent extent of your primary cancer growth by taking a careful history of your symptons, examining you clinically and arranging, with your agreement, whatever tests—X-rays, scans, blood tests and so on—are necessary to provide a complete picture.

Once it is concluded that complete removal of the primary cancer growth, together with a margin of apparently normal tissues, is feasible, it is then important to check for any evidence of secondary growths. Lymphatic spread can be looked for by feeling the appropriate lymph node areas if they are close to the surface, or by checking them by special X-rays (as described in Chapter 4) if they are deep-seated. What follows refers just to the lymph nodes that drain the site of your primary cancer growth. If these lymph nodes are enlarged, the cancer has probably spread to them. However, groups of cancer cells can also be present in normal sized nodes. The only way of being quite sure whether or not a node is involved is to examine it under the microscope. Of course, this can only be done if the node is removed. Therefore, if you have a type of cancer which often spreads through the lymph system, your surgeon will probably recommend removal of the nodes which drain the primary cancer site, even if these nodes are normal in size. Their removal will certainly be recommended if they are enlarged unless they are attached to nearby tissues, such as the overlying skin, indicating that the cancer is not confined within the nodes themselves. Complete removal is rarely possible if this has happened.

Cancer can almost never be cured by surgery once it has spread through the bloodstream. Before agreeing to surgery aimed at curing you, make sure that the likely spots for blood-borne secondary deposits have been checked. Different cancers tend to spread to different organs. For each type there is a typical pattern which your doctor should know. The likely spots should be checked by taking a history of your symptoms, examining you and arranging tests such as blood tests, X-rays and scans. For example, if your cancer tends to spread to the lung, at the very least your doctor should ask you directly whether you have a cough with or without blood in the sputum, shortness of breath or chest pain. Whether or not you have these symptoms, your lungs should be examined and you should have a plain chest X-ray. Sometimes, the search should be more thorough than this, especially if very extensive surgery is planned with the sole aim of curing you. I am referring here to surgery that is so drastic that, if you are *not* cured, you stand to gain absolutely nothing or even to be worse off.

For example, some surgeons recommend very major surgery for locally extensive cancer of the cervix (neck of the womb). This operation is sometimes recommended for cancer of the cervix that has grown into nearby pelvic organs: removal of the entire womb, upper vagina, fallopian tubes, both ovaries, all pelvic lymph nodes, the bladder and the lower bowel. The woman is left with bags on openings in the abdominal wall for both urine and faeces. People who agree to such surgery *only* because it gives them a chance of being cured altogether, should be checked very, very carefully for blood-borne secondary deposits beforehand. The check on the lungs I described above would not be sufficient if surgery like this was planned. Because the lungs are a common site for secondary cancer of the cervix they should be checked with a CT scan before such a drastic operation.

On the other hand, some of the less drastic operations aimed at cure also have a secondary aim. Surgical removal can be the best way of preventing or relieving symptoms from the primary growth. Thus, even people who are not cured may stand to gain something important from these operations—prevention or relief of unpleasant symptoms. Find out whether this is true for the operation that has been recommended for you. If you are sure that the operation is worth having even if if doesn't cure you, it doesn't matter so much if small secondary deposits are not found before the operation. Finding them *after* the operation like this would certainly be disappointing, but just think how much worse it would be for a patient who had had the operation for cervix cancer described above—it would be a complete tragedy.

Surgical Treatment of Secondary Growths

What part can surgery play in the treatment of cancer which has already formed secondary growths? As we have seen, if the cancer has only spread to the lymph nodes which drain the primary cancer site, it may still be cured simply by removal of both the primary growth and the involved group of nodes. With some particular types of cancer, the chance of cure is improved if chemotherapy or radiotherapy is used as well as surgery, but surgery alone *can* cure some of these people.

What if the cancer has spread further—either through the blood or more extensively through the lymph system? Most of these people cannot be cured by any form of treatment. The exceptions are those who have one of the few types of cancer which are extremely sensitive to either radiotherapy or chemotherapy. The chances of curing *these* people may be improved by combining surgical removal of the primary growth, and sometimes also of large secondary growths, with chemotherapy or radiotherapy. However, surgery on its own cannot cure any of them. Some of the cancers which can be cured by such combined treatments are cancers of the testis (both seminomas and non-seminomateous germ cell tumours), ovary, kidney (Wilm's tumour), muscle (rhabdomyosarcoma) and bone (osteogenic sarcoma).

Why is surgery recommended at all for extensive cases of these types of cancer if they are so sensitive to chemotherapy or radiotherapy? Basically the chance of chemotherapy or radiotherapy completely eradicating every cancer cell depends very much on the number of cancer cells there are to start with. It also depends on the size of the individual growths. Surgery can improve the chances of cure by reducing the number and size of cancer growths. The fewer cells there are to start with, the less likely that some of them will be resistant to the chemotherapy or radiotherapy treatment. The smaller the individual cancer growths, the less likely that the cancer cells in the middle of them will escape being killed by the chemotherapy or radiotherapy. Cancer cells can escape being killed by these treatments if they are situated where there is a poor blood supply and very little oxygen—conditions which occur in the middle of large tumour growths.

Occasionally surgeons recommend the removal of blood-borne secondary cancer growths when the cancer is one that is *not* sensitive to chemotherapy or radiotherapy treatment. The chance of being cured in these circumstances is minute. Blood-borne secondary deposits are usually multiple. The very fact that one is detected is proof that cancer cells have been in the bloodstream and are likely to be lying hidden in tiny clumps in other parts of the body. Simply removing detectable blood-borne secondary deposits without doing anything else is very unlikely to cure any cancer.

There is one very special set of circumstances where removal of secondary growths may produce a long remission, although very rarely a cure. These are the conditions. There should be no more than two or three secondary growths. They should have appeared a long time, several years at least, after treatment of the primary. They should be proved to be slow growing by observation over several months. These conditions very rarely occur. Examples I have seen include melanoma, Grawitz tumours (kidney) and slow growing soft tissue sarcomas.

Weighing Cost Against Benefit

Say you have a cancer that fulfills all the conditions I have described—one for which cure by surgical removal seems possible. Perhaps you are prepared to pay any price at all for any chance at all of cure. If not, you still need to weigh the likely benefit against the likely cost before agreeing to the operation.

Check the questions I listed at the beginning of this chapter. What is the chance of cure? What other ways, if any, are there of achieving a cure? Some cancers which can be cured by surgical removal can also be cured by radiation treatment. Surgery has certain advantages—diseased tissues are actually seen, removed and examined under the microscope for completeness of removal. There is no equivalent way of being sure that radiation treatment includes the whole of the primary cancer. Surgery takes a few hours and a week or two in hospital, radiation treatment can take six to eight weeks. On the other hand, radiation treatment can be less mutiliating. For example, patients with cancers of the tongue, lip, throat, larynx (voice-box) and breast are likely to be much less disfigured if treated with radiotherapy than if treated with surgery.

Ask whether your chances would be improved by combining

surgery with other forms of treatment. Radiotherapy and chemotherapy are very specialised types of treatment so your surgeon will probably not know a lot about them. Ask to be referred to these specialists if you suspect or know that they could play a useful part in your treatment.

Make sure you have answers to *all* of the questions at the beginning of this chapter before making your decision. Surgery aimed at curing cancer should not be rushed into but, rather, carefully planned. This means there should be plenty of time to get all the information you need.

Consider every aspect of the possible 'cost' and benefit that is important to *you*, not just what your surgeon accepts as important. *You* are the one who will be stuck with any disfigurement, discomfort or inconvenience, *not* your surgeon! Anything *you* think is important, *is* important. Don't be talked out of what you know about yourself.

After The Operation

What does your surgeon mean when he or she says: 'I think I've got it all?' This expression is unfortunately often used — unfortunately because it is so misleading. I'm not sure whether surgeons say this *knowing* it is misleading or whether they simply don't realise that most patients take it to mean that they have definitely been cured by the operation. What I do know is that, if it is said to you, you should ask exactly what is meant. It is certainly *not* a guarantee of cure. It is sometimes even said when the surgeon knows that cure is not possible!

If your surgeon says this within a day or two of the operation, it means only that he or she has removed all the cancer that was detected before and/or visible during the operation. If your surgeon says it after receiving the pathology report, it probably means that, when it was examined under the microscope, cancer cells were not seen extending right out to the edge of the removed tissue.

The fact of the matter, as you and I know, is that *no one* can be sure that no cancer remains in your body immediately after an operation. You can only be sure that this *was* true, after enough time has gone by for any remaining seedlings to activate and form detectable tumours.

Just as you should insist on getting the results of any tests you have, so you should make sure that your doctor tells you exactly what was found at the operation, and what procedure was done. Ask what the pathologist found when the removed tissues were examined under the microscope. Ask what all these facts mean for you. Here is a chance which you should not miss to obtain definite and useful information about your own particular case. Now that all the details are known your doctor should be able to give you more accurate information about what to expect in the future and what further treatment, if any, should be considered. You can only make the best plans and decisions for yourself if you get this information.

Say, for example, you have had a breast removed. You have been told it was the common type of breast cancer — an adenocarcinoma. If it was confined completely to the breast, the chance of cure is about two in three. If it has spread to the lymph nodes in the armpit, the chance of cure is about one in three, even less if many of the nodes were affected. The chance is possibly improved by having some chemotherapy as well as the surgery. If it had grown into the nearby skin or muscle, or spread to the nodes in the neck, there is only a tiny chance of complete and permanent cure, whatever treatment is used. Before your operation you would not have been sure which of these facts applied to your particular case. After your operation you can be sure.

The exact figures are different for different cancers, but they all tend the same way. The outlook is best if it is confined to the organ it started in. It is less good if it has spread to the nearest lymph glands. It is even less good if it has spread into adjacent tissues. It is worst of all if it has spread through the blood, in which case hopefully an operation aiming at cure would not have been attempted. Ask your surgeon for the figures which apply in your particular case.

I know I'm asking you to be very brave here. It may seem much easier to say: 'Well, I'll just hope for the best—I don't want to know what my chances are.' Don't forget you can still hope for the best when you *do* know what your chances are! There are disadvantages to being ignorant. It can mean that you miss out on having additional treatment which might improve your chances. It also means that you cannot realistically plan your personal life. I feel very sad when I remember how often people who have been referred to me for extensive cancer have said things like this: 'My surgeon told me three years ago that he'd got it all. I've just kept on leading a normal life. If only I'd known this was likely to happen I would have . . . taken that overseas trip I've planned for so long . . . left that job I hated so much and gone back to studying . . . made up with my brother-in-law so I could see more of my sister . . . learnt to drive a car . . . left my husband then instead of waiting till the kids were older . . .'

Perhaps these people would have made the same decisions if they had known the true situation. Perhaps not. Be brave and ask the questions I suggest. Then, you can make decisions about your personal life which do take into account what is likely to happen in the future. Try to keep this information in perspective. Some people go to extremes—they either allow themselves to be overwhelmed by it or they dismiss it from their minds altogether. Remember that, whatever the statistics say, you can still *hope* that you will be the lucky exception. Most of us thrive on hope and why not? Just try not to let that hope develop into a fixed and unrealistic belief that you *will* be the exception. Such a belief could prevent you from making the most of whatever life you do have left.

SURGERY AIMED AT PREVENTING OR RELIEVING SYMPTOMS

Patients with extensive cancer sometimes have symptoms which can be overcome temporarily by an operation. For example, pain and inability to walk due to a fracture through a cancer deposit in the thigh bone can be corrected by strengthening the bone with a steel pin and plate. Weakness and numbness of the legs due to a cancer deposit pressing on the spinal cord may be reversed by relieving the pressure surgically. Pain and vomiting due to blockage of the bowel can be treated by surgically bypassing the blockage, usually by creating a colostomy.

Before agreeing to this sort of surgery, you need to be very clear about what the proposed operation can and cannot achieve. Firstly, these operations cannot and do not have any effect on the cancer itself. Very little of the cancer is actually removed. If you have extensive cancer before one of these operations, you will still have extensive cancer after it.

Secondly, some of these situations are life threatening, for example, the bowel obstruction. In these situations the operation achieves two things—as well as temporarily getting rid of some symptoms it may also temporarily prolong your life. This is not necessarily a good thing, given that the operation does nothing to change the extent of your disease. Unless you are having treatment which could cure you, you will still die of cancer sooner or later anyway. It is possible that to die sooner of a bowel obstruction could be better than to do so later of some other complication of cancer.

If your situation is *not* life threatening, for example, a broken bone or a spinal cord under pressure, your decision is relatively straightforward. You basically need to find out simply what difference the operation is likely to make to the quality of your life. What chance is there that pain will be relieved? What chance is there that you will be able to walk after the operation? How soon after? How long would you be in hospital? What is your chance of surviving the operation? What will happen if you don't have the operation? Is there any other way of relieving the symptoms?

If your situation *is* life threatening your decision is more difficult. As well as questions like those above you would also need to ask yourself and your doctor: What do I stand to gain and to lose by going through a major operation which is likely to result in me living a bit longer? What could that extra time be like? How much of it is likely to be spent in hospital? What new problems could the cancer cause in that time? What might I die of later if I don't die of bowel obstruction now? Can my present unpleasant symptoms be controlled by some other means if I decide to let nature take its course?

It takes a very courageous person to refuse a temporarily life saving treatment of any sort. This is definitely not 'taking the easy way out' or 'giving up'. Even though it might be best for everybody, including you, such a refusal is never easy. I hope that whenever the time is right for you, you will be realistic, brave and tough enough to say 'No'.

RECONSTRUCTIVE SURGERY

I want to start this section by saying something very blunt. Once you have cancer in any part of your body, there is *no way* that that part can ever be completely normal again. If you have a cancer of the breast, that breast will never be completely normal again, regardless of what treatment you have. If you have cancer of the lip, your lip will never be completely normal again, regardless of what treatment you have. The same is true for every cancer site.

If you are considering reconstructive surgery, make sure you understand very clearly what can be achieved by it. Reconstructive surgery that surgeons are proud of is very disappointing for many patients. You are likely to be disappointed if you don't find out beforehand exactly what sort of result you can expect, both in terms of appearance and of function. Ask to see 'before' and 'after' photos of patients who have had the proposed surgery. Remember that the appearance may be quite different when the part is being used or the position of the body is changed. For example, a reconstructed 'lip' that looks fine at rest may not move normally when you are talking. A reconstructed 'breast' that looks fine when the woman is clothed and standing up may look quite peculiar when she is naked and lying down. Ask exactly where you will be cut and how long the scars will be. For example, many patients asking about breast reconstruction are surprised to find that they will be left with a very long scar on their back. Often the normal breast is reduced in size to make it easier to match the reconstructed one. Ask about the function of the reconstructed part. For example, a reconstructed 'breast' and 'nipple' do not have the same sensitive nerve endings as a normal breast and nipple. Parts of them are likely to actually be numb or tingly. Obviously a reconstructed 'breast' cannot produce milk like a normal breast. Ask whether the reconstructed part will alter with time—can the tissues shrink, for example.

In my experience, the only people who are happy with reconstructive surgery are those who get answers to these questions beforehand *and* accept that the final result will *not* be a normal part. Don't agree to reconstructive surgery unless your aims are realistic.

If you have your breast reconstructed because you want to be able to get dressed each day without having to fiddle with an external breast prosthesis, you may be very happy with the results of reconstructive surgery. If you have your breast reconstructed because you want to feel and look completely normal, you will certainly be disappointed.

Well, that has covered some of the important things you need to know about surgery—the type of treatment that is usually considered first for cancer. What other treatments may be recommended instead of, or after, surgery? Let's look at radiation treatment next.

Chapter 8

RADIATION TREATMENT

Radiation treatment, when used on its own, is capable of completely curing certain types of cancer. When combined with surgery and/or chemotherapy it can make the cure of some types of cancer more likely than if any one of these treatments was used on its own. Given before or after surgical removal of a primary growth, it can reduce the chance of the cancer growing back again in the same place (local recurrence). Another very important use of radiation is in extensive cancer, where it can contribute greatly to the relief of symptoms.

Clearly radiation is a valuable form of cancer treatment. Just what is it then, and what are its limitations?

WHAT IS RADIATION TREATMENT?

The expressions radiation treatment and radiotherapy mean the same thing: treatment with various forms of ionising radiation. The treatment is usually given by beaming the rays through the body from a machine which looks a bit like the ones they take X-rays with. Less commonly, radiation treatment is given by temporarily placing radioactive substances inside the body.

Ionising radiation is radiation that can break molecules into electrically charged particles called ions. Radiation passing through you from a machine outside the body does *not* make you radioactive. If your treatment involved putting radioactive substances in or on your body this would make you temporarily radioactive, but only for as long as the substance was actually present. As soon as it was removed or lost its radioactivity you would no longer be radioactive and it would be perfectly safe for anyone to come into close contact with you.

All forms of ionising radiation are invisible, travel in straight lines, can pass through the body painlessly and are capable of damaging all living cells. Radiation treatment does not burn you. You don't feel anything while it is actually passing through you. X-rays are one form of ionising radiation. For treating cancer very, very much stronger (higher voltage) X-rays are used than for taking X-ray pictures for diagnosis. Other forms of radiation are also used to treat cancer—these are all closely related to X-rays.

WHAT DOES RADIATION DO TO HUMAN CELLS?

Ionising radiation is harmful to all human cells—both normal and cancerous. You will remember that, because cancer cells are simply a 'disobedient' form of our own body cells, there is no type of treatment that can kill them without harming some of our normal cells. Radiation treatment is no exception to this rule.

Thus, it is never possible to destroy cancer deposits with radiation without injuring nearby normal tissues. This means that radiotherapists are faced with the same challenge every time they plan a person's treatment—how to produce the greatest possible damage to the cancer growths without risking dangerous or otherwise very serious reactions in the normal tissues. In meeting this challenge, they firstly exploit those differences between cancer and normal tissues which make the cancer, on average, more vulnerable to the harmful effects of radiation. Secondly, they plan the treatment so that the cancer cells receive a higher dose than any normal cells and so that tissues which can give rise to dangerous or otherwise serious reactions receive a smaller dose than tissues whose reactions are less troublesome.

Why Radiation Affects Cancer Cells More Than Normal Cells

Greater Proportion of Dividing Cells

Let's now see what makes cancer cells more likely to be killed by radiation than normal cells. Firstly, the part of the cell that is most sensitive to radiation is the part that controls reproduction. This means that tissues with a high proportion of cells that divide frequently show the harmful effects of radiation more obviously and more quickly than tissues in which the cells rarely divide. Cells that are actually in the process of dividing when radiation passes through them are so sensitive to its harmful effects that they die within a few hours. Cells which are not actually dividing at the time of treatment still suffer serious damage to their reproductive ability. They can often continue to function quite normally provided they don't try to divide. Once they do, it is likely that they will die in the attempt. Most cancers have a higher proportion of cells that divide regularly than most normal tissues. Most, but not all, cancers are therefore likely to show more rapid and severe damage after radiation than most, but not all, normal tissues.

Low doses of radiation interfere with the ability of the cell to divide. Higher doses kill cells directly. Therefore any cell can be killed by radiation if the dose is high enough.

It is important to realise how long the delay between treatment and cell death can be. Very rapidly growing tumours may start to shrink within a week or so of starting treatment because their cells divide every few days. On the other hand, the cells of slowly growing tumours only divide every few months. This means that a slowly growing tumour can keep shrinking for some months after radiation is finished.

A delay before radiation damage becomes obvious also occurs with normal cells. For example, the cells lining the mouth divide every day or so, cells on the skin surface every week or so. When radiation is stopped, a reaction in the mouth will quickly start getting better but a skin reaction can keep getting worse for a week or more. The longest delay is seen in the case of tissues whose cells very rarely divide other than when the tissue is injured. These tissues may look fairly normal and function fairly normally for years, but heal very slowly or not at all if they are injured or infected. This poor healing is only partly due to the fact that some of the cells die when they try to divide. Another reason is that blood and lymph vessels are also damaged by radiation leaving tissues with a poor blood supply and sluggish drainage.

Radiation damage to the reproductive ability of cells has one other possible serious consequence. This one is only of concern to those of you who are lucky enough to be cured, or at least to live many years after your treatment. People who have had radiation treatment have a higher than normal, but still small, risk of developing a completely new cancer within the irradiated areas. I am not referring here to a recurrence of the original cancer but to a completely new cancer caused by the radiation. Radiation-caused leukaemia typically develops about five years after radiation. Other types of cancer take twenty or more years. The risk is *small* but definite. When weighing up your cost/benefit balance, do try to keep this one in perspective. I stress that it will only concern you if your treatment is successful in controlling your original cancer.

Ability of Normal Tissues to Repair Injuries

Another major reason for the fact that most cancer growths finish up being more seriously damaged by radiation than most normal tissues is that normal tissues are better at repairing injuries. However normal tissues are injured— whether by cutting, burning, infection, radiation or anything else— they get to work and repair the damage. Repair processes are stimulated by chemicals produced at the site of injury. Cancer cells, having escaped the body's normal controls over division of cells, are not stimulated to divide by these chemicals. Thus, during breaks between radiation treatments, normal tissues are busy repairing the damage while tumours are not.

Repair of normal tissues is carried out partly by division of the cells within the damaged area. In addition, some types of normal cells migrate into the damaged area from other parts of the body. There is no equivalent form of help available for tumours.

While it is true that normal tissues are generally able to repair radiation damage better than tumours, there is a limit to their ability to do this. You know this from experience with other types of injuries. Let us take a simple example. A skin scratch can heal without leaving any mark. A small cut may heal without any help, leaving a small scar. A larger cut may only heal with the help of stitches. If a big chunk of skin and underlying tissues is actually removed, the defect may never heal over without grafting. The eventual appearance and function of an injured tissue depends on how severe the injury was.

In the same way, the eventual state of tissues that have been irradiated depends on how badly they were damaged. This, in turn, depends on the type and dose of radiation and just how it was given. Let us again use skin as an example. After a small dose of radiation, skin can look normal and function normally. After a larger dose it may be thinner than normal, look tightly stretched, move less freely, be darker in colour, have less hairs than before and remain dry when hot. In general, more specialised structures (like hair follicles and sweat glands) are less likely to be restored to normal than less specialised structures after an injury of any sort. Many of the specialised cells are replaced by scar tissue, rather than the original type of cell. Thus the processes of repair do not produce skin which looks or feels completely normal. Neither is irradiated skin completely normal in its ability to respond to further injury, as we have seen. However, unless it has received very high doses, irradiated skin does serve its main purpose of providing a protective covering for the body. On the other hand, after very high doses of radiation, the damage can be so severe that no healing is possible and the skin is lost. An ulcer then forms—one which will never heal without grafting. Naturally, your radiotherapist will be very careful to try to prevent such a serious reaction as this.

The same principles apply for other tissues. For each one, it is known how much radiation can be given on average, without causing damage that cannot be satisfactorily repaired. What is 'satisfactory' is different for different tissues, partly because the loss of specialised structures is more serious for some tissues than others. For example, it is much less serious to have an area of skin which is hairless and can't sweat than to have a kidney which doesn't work.

To summarise this section, then, there are two facts which tend to make cancer by its very nature more vulnerable to radiation than normal tissues. One is that the part of the cell that is most easily damaged by radiation is the part to do with reproduction. The other is that cancer cells cannot repair damage while normal tissues can.

WHY CAN'T WE CURE ALL CANCER WITH RADIATION?

I have already said that any cell can be killed by radiation, provided the dose is high enough. So, what is it that prevents us from using radiation to cure all people with cancer?

Radiation is a Local Treatment

The first problem is that radiation (with a few exceptions which I will mention later) is, like surgery, a *local* form of treatment. Only known cancer deposits, or areas that are very likely to be involved, are treated. This means that any undetected groups of cancer cells lying outside the irradiated area escape treatment. The treatment then cannot cure the patient, not because it fails to kill the treated cells, but because some cells are not treated at all. It is exactly the same sort of problem as we have with surgery that is aimed at cure. Careful assessment reduces the chance of some cancer escaping untreated. However, as you know, there are no tests that are capable of picking up very tiny groups of cancer cells. This means that even the most careful search for secondaries followed by a course of treatment which kills every cancer cell in the treated area cannot be guaranteed to produce a complete and permanent cure.

The Reaction of Normal Tissue Limits the Safe Dose

Even if we could reliably locate every cancer cell, it would still not be possible to cure every cancer by radiation treatment. This is basically because the reactions of the normal tissues force us to limit doses to a level which cannot cure some cancers. Whether or not a cancer can be cured depends on its location, size, and type, and the general conditions of the patient.

The location is important for two reasons. Firstly, a cancer located in or near tissues which give rise to dangerous or otherwise severe radiation reactions cannot safely be given the same dose as one in a less critical location. Secondly, cancers whose cells look exactly the same under the microscope have different chances of being cured by radiation depending on where in the body they started. The reasons for this are not really understood but it is a fact that should be taken into account by your radiotherapist when planning a treatment. For example, a cancer starting just above the voice-box is less likely to be cured by radiation than exactly the same type of cancer starting in the vocal cords.

Why is the size an important guide as to whether or not a cancer is likely to be cured? One reason is that, because bigger cancers contain more cells, the chance that they will contain some cells which have a natural resistance to radiation is higher than for small cancers. Another reason is that tumours generally do not develop an efficient blood supply. This means that big tumours contain a high proportion of cells which are getting very little oxygen. This is important because cells which are getting very little oxygen are not as sensitive to radiation as cells which are getting plenty of oxygen. It takes two to three times the dose of radiation to kill the poorly oxygenated cells. A third reason is that big growths contain a higher proportion of cells which are not actively dividing than small growths. As we have seen, cells which are not dividing are less sensitive to radiation.

The bigger the tumour, the more of these relatively resistant cells it will contain. However, some of them are present even in tumours that are only a few millimetres across. The chances of curing growths which contain some poorly oxygenated cells and some cells which are not dividing can be improved by giving the radiation treatment in small doses spread over some weeks rather than giving the whole dose in one treatment session. As the cancer shrinks, cells which were not dividing start to divide and cells which were poorly oxygenated get more oxygen. Thus, as the weeks go by, these cells become much more sensitive to radiation treatment than they were to start with. Although the results are better when the treatment is spread out like this, bigger cancers still need a much higher total dose. Even with a higher dose, there is still a much smaller chance of curing the bigger cancers. Very big cancers simply cannot be cured with doses that are safe.

As an example, let's take the situation with secondary deposits from cancer of the mouth in lymph nodes in the neck. When the lymph nodes are 4–6cm in diameter, the dose needed to eradicate the cancer is about half as much again as when the secondary deposits are so small that the nodes are normal in size. In spite of the higher dose, the enlarged nodes are also much less likely to be cleared. Nodes bigger than 6cm cannot be cleared of cancer with a safe dose of radiation. The dose that would be needed would completely destroy some of the surrounding normal tissues. The alternative of surgical removal of such big glands is likely to be a better option than radiation. This is not the same as saying that a safe dose of radiation would be useless. It could shrink such big nodes temporarily but would be very unlikely to cure the cancer altogether. In fact, it is generally true that the dose needed to temporarily control symptoms is much less than the dose needed to completely destroy a cancer deposit. Therefore it is often possible to safely control symptoms by radiation when it would not be possible to cure the cancer by it.

Just as the average dose that is safe for each normal tissue is known, so the average dose that will destroy each type of cancer is known. Some types of cancer are more sensitive than others. For example, one type of cancer of the testis—seminoma—is much more likely to be cured by radiation than other types of testicular cancer. On average, lymphoma in lymph nodes is more sensitive to radiation than secondary cancer in lymph nodes. Ewing's sarcoma of bone is much more sensitive to radiation than other primary bone cancers. Thus the type of cancer is important in predicting whether it is likely to be cured by radiation and what dose will probably be necessary.

Don't forget that the average doses that can safely be given and the average doses that will destroy particular types of cancer are just that: average. They are not doses which can be guaranteed to produce the same result in every person. Some people's tumours are less sensitive than average. Some patients' tissues are more sensitive than average. This means that radiation fails to cure some people of cancers which are usually curable. Sometimes this is simply because their tumour is less sensitive than average — a dose that would cure most people is not effective. Sometimes it is because the usual dose cannot safely be given because the person's tissues cannot take it.

On the whole, healthy tissues can take more radiation than tissues that are scarred, infected or otherwise diseased. As a rule, the tissues of older people can take less radiation than those of younger people, because they tend to have less ability to heal, a poorer blood supply and so on. Tissues that have previously been exposed to the average safe dose of radiation can never safely be re-treated, not even many years later, because the effects of radiation are permanent. Some chemotherapy drugs increase the sensitivity of some normal tissues to radiation. A dose of radiation that is normally safe can produce some serious reactions in people having these particular drugs. Thus there are many factors which can make a usually effective and safe dose of radiation unsafe for some individuals. These should all be considered by your radiotherapist when treatment is planned.

WHAT BENEFITS CAN BE ACHIEVED WITH RADIATION TREATMENT?

Read this section very carefully. I strongly recommend that you make sure that you discuss your case with a radiotherapist (specialist in radiation treatment) before making a treatment decision if any of the following circumstances apply to you. The first is the easiest: when your doctor recommends radiation. In this case there will be no problem about getting a referral! However, there are also other circumstances where I believe you would be wise to insist on referral to a radiotherapist, even if your doctor objects. Firstly, if you have a type of cancer which is listed here as being very sensitive to radiation. Secondly, if you believe that any of the situations described here where radiation *can* play a useful part apply to you. Thirdly, if you have any other reason to believe that radiation treatment could help you—say, from talking with other people with cancer, friends or hospital staff or from something else you have read.

Radiation treatment is highly specialised. The person who can give you the most accurate description of the part that radiation could play in your treatment is a radiotherapy specialist. A radiotherapist is much more likely than other doctors to know exactly what results *could* be achieved and what the side effects are really likely to be. You have the right to have the opportunity to ask questions of a specialist who knows the answers. Don't be fobbed off by any other doctor who dismisses your request for a referral with a statement like: 'It would do you more harm than good' or 'If *I* thought you should have it, I would already have referred you'.

Remember that the reason to insist on a referral is not that you *know* you should have radiation treatment. It is that you suspect it *might* help you. After discussing your case with the radiotherapist, you may decide that you don't want to have radiation treatment. Don't be embarrassed if this is your decision. It doesn't mean that you were wrong to insist on the referral. Seeing a specialist gives you a better chance of obtaining the reliable and accurate information that you need to make the best possible decision.

Cure Of Cancer

There are some types of cancer which can be cured by radiation alone, unassisted by any other form of treatment. These include cancers of the skin (squamous cell and basal cell types), lip, tongue, lining of the mouth, tonsil, salivary glands, sinuses, back of the throat, larynx (voice-box), back of the eye (retinoblastoma), thyroid gland, oesophagus (gullet), breast, bladder, prostate gland, cervix (neck of the womb), uterus (womb), bone (giant cell tumours, Ewing's sarcoma), brain (medulloblastoma) and lymph nodes (Hodgkin's disease and some types of non-Hodgkin's lymphoma). Lymphomas starting in other organs can also be cured by radiation. Radiation is also very useful for controlling the symptoms of these types of cancer. In this section we will be discussing only radiation used with the aim of cure (see pages 188–89 for symptom control).

Please understand that I am *not* saying that radiation is always the 'best' way of trying to cure these types of cancer. Neither am I saying that radiation can cure every person with cancer of these types. Far from it. I am simply saying that radiation should always be *considered* for them. Whether or not it is the 'best' treatment for you depends on how its likely cost and benefit compare to the likely cost and benefit of other possible treatments in your particular case.

Considering Alternatives

You should consider each of the possible treatments separately and combined when making your decision. For example, you could decide that radiation plus surgery, or radiation plus chemotherapy, is better than either treatment alone. Alternatively you may decide that the extra benefit likely to be gained by combining two treatments is too small to warrant the additional likely cost. Don't forget that your doctor is likely to recommend the treatment which has the best chance of curing you, whatever the likely 'cost'. *You* need to know about all aspects of the possible cost before deciding whether this is the treatment that is best for you. For example, for many people the likely eventual appearance and function of the involved part are easily as important as the cure rate. In general, one of the major advantages that radiation has over surgery is that it produces a less drastic change in appearance and function. This is not a hard-and-fast rule—there are exceptions to it. You need to find out what applies in your particular case.

Don't be embarrassed to tell your doctor that the final appearance

and function are important in deciding which treatment is best
for you. You're the one who has to live with it. You can ask to see
'before' and 'after' photos of people who have been treated by
each method. You might prefer a treatment that will alter your
appearance less even though it has a smaller chance of curing you.
That is fine as long as you understand that a treatment that is less
likely to cure you is also less likely to prevent the cancer from
growing back again in the same place (local recurrence). Such a
local recurrence could be disfiguring, uncomfortable and difficult
to treat. Ask how likely this is to happen with each treatment and
how it could be treated if it does. Take this information into
account when making your decision.

Here are a few examples of the sorts of situation you could be
faced with.

Early cancers of the larynx (voice-box) are equally likely to be
cured by radiation as by removal of the larynx. Radiation has the
very great advantage of preserving the ability to talk. However,
more advanced cancers have a better chance of being cured if they
are removed. If this applies in your case you will have to balance
the benefit of a higher cure rate against the disadvantage of loss of
the voice-box when deciding which treatment to have.

A small retinoblastoma has an equal chance of being cured
either by radiation or by removal of the eye. Radiation is clearly
preferable if it can preserve vision. This is sometimes possible
when the tumour is small and suitably located. On the other
hand, if vision is going to be lost anyway, it could be better to
remove the eye, because an artificial eye is likely to look better
than an irradiated one.

The chances of living five years without any cancer recurrence
is the same when a *small* breast cancer lump is removed and the
breast irradiated as when the patient has a mastectomy (removal
of the breast). It is also very likely that the eventual cure rates are
the same, although this has not definitely been proven. If you
have breast cancer and don't wish to have a mastectomy, insist on
your right to discuss your case with a radiotherapy specialist.
This will give you the best chance of finding out what facts and
figures apply in your particular case before making a decision.

Let's look at some other considerations which may influence

your choice when it comes to deciding between radiation and other forms of treatment. Factors which can influence the likely cost and benefit include size, location, extent and exact type of cancer as determined by microscopic examination.

Size of Cancer

I have already explained that small cancers are much more likely to be cured by radiation than large ones, and that a lower dose is needed for smaller growths. Even if you have one of the radio-sensitive types of cancer listed above, radiation may not be the best form of treatment if it is large. The likely side effects of the high dose that would be needed could make surgery a better alternative. In fact, radiation used on its own may not even be a realistic alternative. It simply may not be possible to cure your cancer by radiation without producing very serious or life-threatening complications.

Location of Cancer

This depends to some extent on the next factor—the location of the cancer. If it is in or near tissues which can give rise to particularly dangerous or unpleasant radiation reactions, the safe dose of radiation will be less than if it is in a less critical location. The location may determine whether radiation or surgery is the better choice.

Extent of Cancer

The extent of the cancer is the next factor to consider. We have already seen that a major drawback of both surgery and radiation is that they are local forms of treatment. For most of the cancers listed at the beginning of this section, radiation alone can produce a cure only if the cancer is confined to the primary site and the nearby lymph nodes. Another requirement for curability, as we have seen, is that each of the growths must be quite small.

Type of Cancer

Lymphomas warrant a separate mention because they don't spread in the same way as most tumours. Hodgkin's disease *can* be cured by radiation provided it is present only in lymph nodes and the spleen. If it involves other organs such as the liver, bone marrow, or lungs, it can only be cured by chemotherapy. This is not to say that radiation is always the best choice of treatment even for Hodgkin's disease that involves only lymph nodes and spleen. In some such cases, chemotherapy has a higher chance of producing a cure. The chances of cure by each method depend on the type of Hodgkin's disease (there are four different types under the microscope), whether or not you have symptoms like fever and weight loss, how big the nodes are and where they are located. If you have Hodgkin's disease, ask about the likely benefit and the likely cost of having either radiation or chemotherapy or both together. You may not be told that there is an alternative unless you ask directly. By the way, surgical removal of the involved nodes is *not* an effective form of treatment in Hodgkin's disease. Surgical biopsy is necessary to make a diagnosis. Surgical exploration may also be recommended in order to assess the extent of the disease. In neither case is the surgery actually a form of treatment. Hodgkin's disease cannot be cured by surgery.

Certain types of non-Hodgkin's lymphoma can also be cured by radiation provided they are localised to one or two groups of lymph nodes. Again, in some cases, the chance of cure would be higher with chemotherapy. Make sure you find out all about each treatment from someone who is experienced in its use before making a decision. As in many situations, your doctor may decide which treatment is 'best' without discussing it with you or offering you any options. In this case you will have to ask directly for the alternatives. You might also have to insist on referral to the appropriate specialist in order to get the information you need.

Certain types of thyroid cancer (well differentiated papillary and follicular types) can be cured by a unique radiotherapeutic method, even when they have spread through the bloodstream. It is not even necessary to know where the secondary deposits are! How is this done? The method relies on the fact that well differentiated thyroid cancers have not lost the ability to concentrate iodine in their cells. Normal thyroid tissue takes iodine out of the blood in order to make thyroid hormone. Although they can't make thyroid hormone with it, the above-named well differentiated types of thyroid cancer also extract iodine from the blood. This ability is exploited by giving the patient a radioactive form of iodine. Provided all of the normal thyroid gland has been removed or destroyed by a previous dose of radioactive iodine, the radioactive iodine concentrates in the cancer cells. They therefore receive a very high dose of radiation, which has a very good chance of destroying them completely. The rest of the body receives very little radiation, so the side effects of this treatment are mild. There have been many attempts to find radioactive substances which would be concentrated in other types of cancer cells, so far with no real success.

Going back to external radiation, the exact type of cancer as determined by examination of a sample under the microscope is also important in determining the dose that would probably be needed and the chance that this would produce a cure. One reason is that some types of cancer are more sensitive to radiation than others. For example, a type which typically has a large proportion of actively dividing cells will be more sensitive than one with many dormant cells. The other reason is that some types of cancer are much more likely to spread through the bloodstream than others. Because radiation is a local form of treatment, it has less chance of curing cancers which tend to spread very early in the course of the disease.

As with every form of treatment which aims for cure, it is many years before you can be sure that treatment was completely successful. The initial aim is to achieve a complete remission, because of course only complete remissions can eventually prove to be complete cures. I have explained that an irradiated cancer can keep shrinking for some months after completion of treatment. This means that you may have to wait before even being sure that you are in complete remission. Ask your doctor how long you must wait before you can be fairly confident that recurrence will not occur. The time is different for different types of cancer.

Cure Of Cancer By Combinations Of Treatment Which Include Radiation

Radiation can be combined with other forms of treatment to

produce cure rates which are greater than when any one treatment is used on its own. The radiation may be to the primary site or to likely or definite secondary sites.

Ependymoma, and low grade astrocytoma are examples of cancers which are more likely to be cured by a combination of surgery and radiation, both to the primary site, than by either surgery or radiation alone. These two examples are both brain cancers which, because of their location, are difficult to remove completely. Radiation given after surgery increases the cure rate by killing any cells which have not been removed. As we will see in the next section, pre- or post-operative radiation to the primary site usually makes a difference only to the chance of local recurrence and not to the chance of complete cure. These cancers are exceptions to this rule because they rarely spread outside of the central nervous system. Effective local treatment therefore has a good chance of curing them completely.

Some cancers which have spread can be cured by removing the primary cancer surgically and irradiating the secondary deposits. The main examples are seminoma (a type of testicular cancer) and dysgerminoma (a rare type of ovarian cancer). The primary cancer is removed mainly in order to make a definite and exact diagnosis. These types of cancer are so sensitive to radiation that even quite large secondary deposits can be destroyed completely using safe doses of radiation. These cancers are also very sensitive to chemotherapy treatment. The chance of cure is greater with chemotherapy than with radiation if the disease is very extensive. However, chemotherapy has more side effects. If you have one of these types of cancer you will have to find out what figures apply in your particular case and exactly what each treatment would involve in order to make the best decision for you.

There are some cancers which are so likely to spread through the bloodstream that it is best to take it for granted that they already have when planning treatment. Combinations of chemotherapy with surgery and/or radiation have a higher chance of curing these types of cancer than any one treatment on its own. These cancers include acute leukaemias, rhabdomyosarcoma (cancer of muscle), Ewing's sarcoma (a cancer of bone), Wilm's tumour (a kidney cancer), and small cell anaplastic cancer of the lung. Chemotherapy is the mainstay of treatment for these types of cancer, because it travels through the blood and gets to nearly every part of the body. However, if local forms of treatment— surgery and radiation—are directed to the areas where cancer cells are most likely to escape being killed by the chemotherapy drugs, the cure rate is higher than if chemotherapy is used on its own.

Where are cancer cells most likely to escape being killed by chemotherapy drugs? Firstly, they may escape wherever there are big deposits. One of the biggest deposits is often, but not always, the primary cancer. There may be a choice between surgery and radiation to tackle these large deposits. Secondly, there are parts of the body where there seems to be some sort of barrier to the penetration of chemotherapy drugs. Radiotherapy can be used to treat these areas. They are the central nervous system (brain and spinal cord), the testis and the ovary. For example, in acute lymphoblastic leukaemia of children, the chance of leukaemia cells getting into the central nervous system, testis or ovary is so high that preventive treatment of these areas by radiation is recommended. This addition to the usual chemotherapy treatment has been shown to improve the cure rate.

Bone marrow transplantation is a special instance where radiation is combined with other treatments to produce some cures. The preparation includes radiation of the whole body. Although bone marrow transplantation has been tried for many types of cancer, the only ones it can cure are certain types of leukaemia. The entire treatment package is very arduous, dangerous and lengthy and the chance of cure is usually not high. Try very hard to get all the facts before agreeing to this type of treatment (see also p 225–26).

Obviously, the more different types of treatment you have, the more your treatment is likely to 'cost'. The situation with combination treatments is so complex that you could be very tempted just to tell your doctor to go ahead with whatever is most likely to cure you. The problem is that doctors have a tendency to overtreat, as we have seen. They are likely to want to add to your treatment anything that could be active against your cancer. They will probably make little or no attempt to weigh the likely additional cost against the likely additional benefit. In any case, you can do that much better than they can. It is therefore very important that you ask exactly what difference *each part* of your treatment is likely to make. What could happen if you only had one type of treatment? Does the addition of radiation improve the cure rate or only the local recurrence rate? How difficult is it to treat a recurrence? Would you still have a chance of cure if the disease recurred or is the 'first bite at the cherry' really your only chance? You will have to try to weigh up the possible costs against the possible benefits to come up with the decision that is best for you.

Prevention Of Local Recurrence

Radiation treatment is often recommended before or after surgical removal of a primary cancer. It is important that you understand what can be gained by doing this.

Firstly, as I mentioned in the previous section, the addition of radiation to surgical removal of a primary cancer very rarely makes any difference to the chance of complete and permanent cure. However, it can make a difference to the chance that cancer will grow back again in the same place—local recurrence.

Radiation *before* an operation may be recommended if you have a large primary cancer that your surgeons feel they cannot completely remove. Their recommendation is based on the hope that shrinking your cancer by radiation could change it from one that is too large and extensive to be removed to one that can be removed completely. The fact is that a cancer that is too extensive to be removed can rarely be cured by any means, unless it is a type that is extremely sensitive to radiation or chemotherapy. It is also a fact that radiation, followed by a less extensive operation than would have been necessary to start with, is an approach that very rarely produces cures. It sounds like a good idea but unfortunately, it doesn't work. I would question the radiotherapist and surgeon very closely indeed before agreeing to such a plan.

Radiation *after* an operation is often recommended when it is either suspected or definitely known that cancer cells have been left behind. You will remember from the chapter on surgery that the chances of not being able to completely remove the cancer can be reduced by careful assessment before the operation. Post-operative radiation is more likely to be recommended after poorly planned than after carefully planned surgery. Radiation in this setting is also very unlikely to improve the cure rate. However, depending on the type and location of the cancer it *can* certainly reduce the chance of local recurrence. If this approach is recommended to you, ask what the chances of local recurrence are with and without radiation. Of course, if your surgeon *knows* that cancer cells are still there, local recurrence is certain if no other treatment is given. Find out how much the chance is likely to be improved by radiation and at what 'cost' to you. Are there any other ways of reducing the chance of local recurrence? Ask what difference it would make if radiation was reserved until the local recurrence occurred, instead of being given as a preventive. Would cure still be possible if you waited until you got a definite local recurrence? What symptoms could a local recurrence cause and how could they be treated? Don't agree to the additional treatment unless you feel sure that the likely benefit is greater than the likely cost.

Treatment Of Symptoms

I believe that one of the most valuable roles of radiation in cancer treatment is palliative— the control of symptoms. Here, the aim is not to cure or completely control the cancer, but simply to treat some of its symptoms. As a rule, the doses needed for palliative treatment are much less than for curative treatment because the aim is only to shrink a particular cancer deposit, not to kill every cell in it. Thus, the side effects of palliative treatment tend to be relatively minor. There are many symptoms that can be relieved *temporarily* by reducing the size of a cancer deposit.

Pain due to a cancer deposit in a bone can often be relieved by radiation. The radiation can also reduce the chance of fracture of the affected bone. Pain due to pressure on nerves or other sensitive structures near a cancer deposit may be relieved by shrinking the growth by radiation. Symptoms due to cancer in the brain like headache, vomiting, paralysis and numbness may be temporarily relieved by radiation treatment. A cancer growth that has ulcerated through the skin may be shrunk sufficiently for the skin to heal over. Bleeding from an ulcerated cancer deposit may be stopped by radiation. A cancer that is causing an obstruction may be shrunk by radiation enough to temporarily relieve the blockage and its symptoms. For example, blockage of blood or lymph vessels, bronchial tubes, the oesophagus (gullet), the ureter (tube from kidney to bladder) or the lower bowel may be temporarily relieved by radiation.

If radiation is recommended to you for control of symptoms, I suggest you read Chapter 6 carefully. Aspects to consider are discussed in detail there. In brief though, the usual cost versus benefit balance must be weighed up. How seriously are the symptoms interfering with your day-to-day life? What other ways are there of treating the symptoms? What exactly would these treatments involve? What chance is there that radiation will control the symptoms? How many treatments would you need? How quickly would it act? Would you have to be hospitalised and if so, for how long? For how long would the symptoms be controlled? How likely is it that the symptom would recur in your lifetime? What side effects of treatment could there be? Could radiation that is mainly aimed at treating a symptom also result in you living longer (for example, by temporarily reducing the size of cancer deposits in the brain or by temporarily opening up an obstructed windpipe)? If it could result in your living longer, is this what you really want? What other symptoms could develop in that extra time? How likely is it that they could be controlled?

These are some of the questions that you should ask yourself and your doctor before deciding whether or not to have palliative radiation treatment.

SOME 'COSTS' OF RADIATION TREATMENT—SIDE EFFECTS

I described briefly on pages 171–75 how our tissues react when they are damaged by radiation. Now let's just see what this means for you in real life—what symptoms can result from those reactions?

These symptoms fall into two distinct groups. There are acute symptoms which occur during or immediately after radiation. There are also delayed symptoms that can occur long after radiation. The severity and nature of both acute and delayed symptoms depend on the type and dose of radiation and on what tissues are irradiated.

Immediate Side Effects Of Radiation

Many of the **immediate** symptoms are due directly to damage to actively dividing cells. There is normally a high proportion of actively dividing cells throughout the linings of the whole intestinal tract from mouth to anus, the whole respiratory tract from nose to bronchial tubes, and the bladder. The skin is another surface which is kept healthy by frequent replacement of its cells with new ones. Radiation stops the normal process of constant renewal of these surfaces.

Thus radiation to the mouth, throat or nose can cause soreness and sometimes ulceration. Radiation to the stomach can cause a vague stomach ache, loss of appetite and nausea. Radiation to the intestines can cause diarrhoea. Radiation to the lungs can cause a dry irritating cough. Radiation to the bladder can cause cystitis— stinging and burning when passing urine and a desire to pass urine frequently. Radiation to the skin can cause redness, soreness and 'peeling'.

It is important to try not to place any extra demands on these areas during radiation. For example, you will be asked not to rub skin that is being radiated, and to avoid tight clothing and hot or cold applications. Steps will be taken to prevent infection in any of these areas— for example, by using antiseptic mouth washes if the mouth is being irradiated. Any infection that does occur must be treated promptly.

The bone marrow is another tissue which normally contains a high proportion of actively dividing cells. However, radiation of part of the bone marrow doesn't usually cause any symptoms provided the rest of the marrow is normal. A large proportion of your active marrow must be irradiated to produce any change in the blood count. Even then, you would be unlikely to experience any symptoms as a result.

The testes and ovaries are also very sensitive to radiation. The ovaries may be irradiated either deliberately, or incidentally when nearby organs are treated. Because they lie within the pelvic cavity it is difficult to shield them from nearby irradiation. The effect depends on the dose. Anything more than very small amounts of radiation is likely to stop menstruation permanently. You would become infertile—unable to have babies. Unless you took replacement hormones, you could experience any of the possible symptoms of a normal menopause, such as hot flushes, relative dryness of the vagina and possibly a loss of interest in sex. If your periods stop, I strongly suggest that you take small doses of female hormones until the usual age of menopause (about fifty) to replace those that would normally be produced by your ovaries. Ask your doctor to prescribe these if they are not offered to you. Read pages 245–46 if you want to learn more about hormone replacement treatment.

The testes, because of their position, are much easier to shield off when nearby areas such as the groin are irradiated. They should receive only a small dose in such cases. If they received a large dose for any reason, they would become small and soft, your libido (interest in sex) would diminish and you would probably become permanently infertile. You might still be able to get an erection and ejaculate (come). However, regular injections of male hormones to replace those normally produced by your testes would probably be needed for normal sexual feelings and function. With or without the hormone injections, your ejaculate would contain very few or no sperm. There is no treatment that could make you fertile.

Most people believe that radiation treatment always causes nausea, and loss of appetite and energy. This is not true. These symptoms are rarely a problem unless large parts of the body are being treated or the treated area includes the abdomen. If the radiation is only to the head, neck, arms or legs, these symptoms would so rarely be due to radiation that another explanation should be looked for.

If you do have nausea, loss of appetite and loss of energy due to radiation, you might find it easier to cope if you keep in mind that they are only immediate reactions. They should disappear within a few days of stopping the treatment. Of these symptoms, only the nausea can be successfully treated (see Chapter 6). There is, however, one way of getting rid of all these symptoms short of completely stopping the radiation. Just reducing the amount of radiation you get each day can eliminate them. This may not be the best thing for you to do in the long run. It would make the whole treatment course last longer and you would need a higher total dose to get the same results. Discuss the situation with your radiotherapist if your symptoms are more than you are prepared to cope with.

A completely different type of immediate reaction is another possible cause of acute symptoms. Due to a reaction to the death of cancer cells, the tumour area sometimes actually swells during the first week or so of treatment. This only causes symptoms if the tumour is critically located. For example, swelling of a brain tumour can temporarily increase the symptoms of high pressure on the brain—nausea, and headache. Swelling of a tumour pressing on the spinal cord can make the pressure symptoms worse. Swelling of a tumour that is partially blocking the windpipe can make breathing more difficult. The swelling lasts only a few days and can be reduced or prevented by the use of a cortisone-like drug (the one used most often is called dexamethasone).

Delayed Side Effects Of Radiation

What about **delayed** reactions to radiation? Here I am referring to reactions occurring months or years after radiation. What symptoms can these reactions cause? The symptoms are caused by loss of specialised cells, formation of scar tissue and damage to blood and lymph vessels. Once they develop, they are permanent. Do you remember my description of delayed skin changes back on page 174? There can be loss of hair and sweat glands. Scar tissue can tighten the skin. Damage to blood and lymph vessels makes the skin less able to cope with further injury such as cutting or infection.

The same sorts of reactions occur in all tissues. Here are some examples. Say the lung is irradiated. The bronchial tubes can lose the ability to produce mucus. Scar tissue can draw in and stiffen the irradiated part of the lung, so that it moves less freely. That part of the lung is more susceptible to infection and less able to handle infection if it does develop.

Say the bladder is irradiated. Scar tissue can draw it in, making it smaller and less flexible. This can result in the need to pass urine in smaller amounts and more often than previously.

Say the spinal cord is irradiated. The nerve cells may be damaged directly or through damage to blood vessels. This can result in tingling or numbness of the legs, even partial or complete paralysis of legs, bowel and bladder (paraplegia).

Radiation-damaged blood vessels become abnormally fragile. Thus some patients who have had part of their bowel or bladder irradiated experience episodes of bleeding from these areas in later years. Both blood and lymph vessels can become narrowed after radiation. This is one of the reasons why irradiated tissues are more susceptible than normal tissues to infection, and also less able to heal further damage of any sort.

As I explained earlier, your radiotherapist knows how much radiation each part of the body can normally take. Your treatment should be planned so that critical areas like the spinal cord do not receive enough radiation to cause serious and permanent consequences. As we have also seen, treatment which has a high chance of curing cancer altogether almost always carries a definite risk of serious and permanent damage to nearby tissues. Ask your radiotherapist directly exactly what risks you would be taking—what changes could occur, what symptoms could result and how likely is this to happen in your particular case?

I mentioned one other type of delayed reaction back on page 173 of this chapter—an increased risk of a new type of cancer developing many years later. There is definitely an increased risk of acute leukaemia after radiation. There is also an increased risk of other types of cancer developing within the treated area. Examples include increased risk of thyroid cancer after the neck has been irradiated, of breast cancer after the breast has been irradiated, of cancer of the womb after the pelvis has been irradiated, and of primary bone cancers in any bone that has been irradiated. Of course, this is a problem only for people whose original treatment was successful in controlling their cancer, and only for a *small* proportion of them.

The doses used to treat symptoms are much less than those needed to cure cancer. This means that both immediate and delayed side effects are rarely serious in the case of palliative treatment. You should still ask your radiotherapist about them however. When the possible benefit is only temporary control of symptoms, you certainly don't want to run the risk of paying a high price in the form of very severe or dangerous side effects.

PLANNING RADIATION TREATMENT

Let's say you have decided to have some radiation treatment. What actually happens next?

First of all, your radiotherapist has to accurately locate the exact area to be treated. He or she must then work out how to get the required dose to that area with the least possible side effects. Care must be taken to ensure that no area of normal tissue receives a dose of radiation that is likely to result in dangerous or otherwise serious side effects.

Planning is assisted by taking special X-rays with a simulator. The simulator is only a machine for taking X-rays, not for treatment. It makes use of the same strength X-rays as does any machine that takes X-ray pictures. Its importance is that it is set up so that the rays from it duplicate exactly the path that the rays from the treatment machine would take. The resulting pictures show exactly what area will be exposed to the much stronger rays from the treatment machine. Both the simulator and the treatment machine are mounted so that they can be moved through a complete circle. The radiotherapist must work out how to position you so that the area to be treated is at the centre of that circle. Then, he or she can be sure that the rays will pass through the area to be treated, regardless of the angle that the machine is at. Once sure of this, the radiotherapist is free to choose the safest angles for treatment. The safest angles are those from which the rays will travel through the least critical tissues on their way to and from the target area.

For example, say the breast, or chest wall after a mastectomy, is to be treated. The ray is beamed in at a glancing angle so that most of it travels only through the skin, muscle and ribs of the chest wall. It is not aimed at right angles to the skin, because then the underlying lung tissues would receive a dose which would be likely to cause permanent scarring.

In general, treatment is very rarely given from one direction only, but rather from a number of angles. In this way, although more normal tissues receive *some* radiation, no one area of normal tissues has the *entire* dose passing through it.

The beams coming from the simulator and treatment machines are rectangular in outline. This shape is suitable for treatment of some areas. If a different shape is required, this is created by changing the shape of the beam before it enters your body. The parts of the beam that are not wanted can be blocked out by metal shields which are designed individually for each patient. The shields are made of a lead alloy through which the rays cannot pass.

As well as the pictures taken by the simulator, your radio-therapist also needs a record of the exact shape of the part of your body that is to be treated. There are various ways of getting an outline of your shape. Once obtained it is transferred to graph paper, on which the area to be treated is also carefully marked. Calculations (often assisted by a computer) are then made to determine exactly what dose of radiation will occur at any particular point in the body. You may be familiar with the lines called isobars on a weather map. These lines connect all points where the same atmospheric pressure was recorded. In the same way isodose curves are drawn on your treatment plan. These lines connect all the points which will receive the same dose of radiation. The calculations and resulting isodose curves may have to be worked out for a number of different treatment plans. The radiotherapist should not be satisfied until a plan is designed which will result in an even dose of the required strength to the target area without a risky dose to any area of normal tissue. If you have a cancer whose type and location are common, it may take only a few hours to finalise your treatment plan because a standard plan which needs only slight adjustments could be used. However, if there is anything unusual about your case, planning could take several days.

It is obvious that these dosage calculations and curves will only be correct provided the positioning of the machine and your body are exactly the same for every treatment. To make this possible, certain key points may be marked on your skin. This is done either with a small tattoo or a marking which must not be washed off before the entire course of treatment is completed. It is essential that you remain perfectly still for the few minutes that it takes to actually give the treatment. Sometimes devices like splints are made to help you to hold the right position. If you are placed in a very uncomfortable or painful position, tell your radiotherapist. Ask whether your treatment plan can be changed so that you can be treated in a more comfortable position.

In most radiotherapy departments, the radiotherapist has a number of treatment machines to choose from. The most suitable machine for a particular patient depends on the location and extent of the area to be treated.

The lowest voltage (strength) machines are used to treat cancers in or very close to the skin. These are also called superficial treatment machines. These rays are at their strongest when they strike the skin and lose strength quite quickly as they pass through the tissues. In the early days of radiation treatment, these were the only machines available. Safe treatment was difficult. To get an effective dose to a deep-seated tumour, a very high dose had to be given to the skin and other tissues lying between the machine and the target area. This is why people who were treated for cancer many years ago were often left with severe scarring.

These days much higher voltage machines have been developed. The high voltage (stronger) rays have a number of advantages. Firstly, they are not absorbed in the same way as they pass through the body. The highest dose occurs *beneath* the skin, not on the skin surface. The stronger (higher voltage) the rays, the deeper does the highest dose occur. Deep-seated cancers can be treated without giving such a high dose to the more superficial tissues. The high voltage rays are also absorbed equally by all tissues, whereas the old low voltage rays were absorbed more by bone than by soft tissues. This uneven absorption made it difficult to work out the exact dose of radiation at any particular point. Another advantage of the higher voltage rays is that they can be focussed much more sharply.

Internal Radiotherapy

As well as having the choice of a number of different machines for beaming rays from *outside* the body, your radiotherapist also has the option of treating some cancers from the *inside*. By positioning a source of radiation (a radioactive substance) actually in or near the cancer, the radiotherapist can concentrate the radiation right where it is wanted. The big advantage over external treatment is that, for the same dose to the surrounding normal tissues, it is possible to get a much bigger dose to the cancer using this method. Such extreme localisation of the treatment can also have its disadvantages however. It can only be fully successful if the cancer is indeed localised to the treatment area. Often the best results can be obtained by combining external and internal forms of treatment.

In some cases, needles containing a radioactive substance are actually put right into the cancer under a general anaesthetic. In other cases, the radioactive substance is placed right next to the cancer. For example, in the treatment of cancer of the cervix an enclosed radioactive substance can be carefully positioned in the vagina. Whenever this sort of treatment is used, the time necessary to deliver the required dose is carefully calculated. This is usually some days. As soon as this time is up the radioactive source is removed. You would be radioactive only while the source was actually in your body. As soon as it was removed you would no longer be radioactive and it would be quite safe for anyone to come into close contact with you.

The time factor is also of vital importance with external radiation. Each treatment is timed exactly to ensure that the correct dose is given.

However radiation is given, the total dose needed depends on how the dose is split up. A certain dose given in a single treatment session has a greater effect than the same dose spread out over many treatments. The effect is greater both on the cancer and on the normal tissues. However, it is usually recommended that treatment is spread out over many treatment sessions. There are a number of good reasons for this, some of which I have already mentioned on pages 176–77. First of all, giving the treatment in small doses separated by breaks gives the normal tissues a chance to repair some of the damage each day. The eventual damage to the normal tissues is therefore less severe than when the whole dose is given in one 'hit'. Secondly, spreading treatment out over some weeks allows more flexibility. As the cancer gets smaller, the size of the area being treated can also be reduced. In this way the radiation to normal tissues can be kept to a minimum. In addition, as we have seen, large cancers have a low proportion of actively dividing cells and a low proportion of well oxygenated cells. This makes them relatively resistant to radiation. Spreading the treatment over a period of weeks allows us to take advantage of the fact that, on average, a cancer becomes more sensitive to radiation as it gets smaller in size.

During the time that you are actually having the radiation, you will be shut in the treatment room on your own. You now know enough about the effects of radiation to understand why no one should be exposed to it unnecessarily. However, the technicians controlling the treatment will be just outside the treatment room. They will be able to both see and hear you and you will be able at least to hear and probably also to see them.

I'm sure that some of the more scientifically minded of you will find out more about radiation. That's fine, but let me say that I don't believe that you need to understand all the technicalities in order to decide whether or not it is the best treatment for you. What you really need to know is what effects it is likely to have on *your* body and on *your* cancer. You don't need to know exactly what it is or exactly what damage it does to atoms, molecules and cells in order to understand what benefits and costs are likely for you if you have it. All you need to be is a real expert on is yourself and you are that anyway!

We have now discussed the two major forms of local cancer treatment. Next we are going to look at some treatments which act throughout the whole body—chemotherapy and hormone treatment.

Chapter 9

CHEMOTHERAPY – GENERAL CONSIDERATIONS

WHAT IS CHEMOTHERAPY?

Chemotherapy is the treatment of cancer by drugs which can disrupt the chemical workings of cells. A wide range of quite different chemicals is covered by the general term 'chemotherapy'. What do these drugs have in common?

How Chemotherapy Works

Firstly, all chemotherapy drugs are capable of damaging or destroying some cancer cells. However, each drug is active only against certain particular types of cancer. When I say active, I mean that it kills *some* of that particular type of cancer cell in *some* patients. There are a few rare types of cancer where there is a high chance of chemotherapy drugs destroying every single cancer cell and so curing the patient. However, for *most* patients for whom chemotherapy is recommended, there is actually no chance of complete cure. Most chemotherapy treatment is aimed only at temporarily reducing the number of cancer cells.

The second feature all chemotherapy drugs share is that they are all systemic treatments. This means they act throughout the body—a big advantage over surgery and radiotherapy, which, as we have seen, are only locally acting treatments. With chemotherapy, it is not necessary to accurately locate every single cancer deposit beforehand. The drugs will get to them anyway, whether we know they are there or not. There are two exceptions to this rule. Cancer cells in the central nervous system (brain, spinal cord and meninges) and the gonads (ovaries and testes) can survive chemotherapy treatment which kills all other cancer cells in the body. There is an invisible barrier which stops the drugs from penetrating efficiently into these parts of the body. Some ways of dealing with this problem are discussed on pages 226–27.

The third fact that is true of all chemotherapy drugs is that they are all capable of damaging or destroying some normal cells. I'm sure this won't surprise you—you already know that cancer cells are just disobedient versions of normal cells. Anything that can damage cancer cells will also damage some normal cells. Chemotherapy drugs are no exception to this rule.

Lastly, all chemotherapy drugs act by disrupting some aspect of the chemical workings of cells. Most drugs interfere in some way or another with the process of cell division. Because of this, cells which divide often are generally the most sensitive to chemotherapy. This is true both for cancerous and for normal cells. Thus, the types of cancer which can be cured by chemotherapy are all rapidly growing ones. The types of normal cells which are most commonly damaged by chemotherapy are the ones that divide often. These include the cells of the lining of the mouth and intestinal tract, the bone marrow and the hair follicles. This is why sore mouth, nausea, vomiting, diarrhoea, low blood counts and loss of hair are common side effects of chemotherapy.

The ability to damage frequently dividing cells is common to most chemotherapy drugs. In addition, certain other types of cells are particularly sensitive to certain drugs. For example, the drug adriamycin can weaken heart muscle cells, bleomycin can cause scarring in the lungs, cis-platinum and high doses of methotrexate can harm the kidneys and vincristine can cause pins and needles and weakness in the arms and legs through damage to the nerves. For each drug, there are also certain types of cancer which tend to be sensitive and other types which tend to be resistant. For each drug that is beyond the research stage, these patterns are well known. It is important to realise that, although they share some features, all chemotherapy drugs are quite different. Find out the names of the particular drugs that are recommended for you, ask your doctor about them and read about them in the next chapter before you make a decision about chemotherapy.

All this means that you can't assume that you will have exactly the same experiences on chemotherapy as anybody else. Different types and stages of cancer are treated with different drugs with different degrees of success. Most chemotherapy treatment is very unpleasant. Most chemotherapy treatment is not capable of permanently curing people. However, there are exceptions to both of these rules. The details of the unpleasantness are different. Some chemotherapy treatment can produce remissions even if it doesn't cure people altogether. Chemotherapy that is useless against some types of cancer can work against other types. You need to find out what the facts are for *your* cancer and the particular chemotherapy drugs recommended for *you*.

BENEFITS OF CHEMOTHERAPY

In order to understand the possible benefits of chemotherapy, we need to know what the possible outcomes of this treatment are. First of all, let us consider those people who have one of the types of cancer which, even after it has spread, *can be cured* by chemotherapy. None of these cancers are common. They include acute lymphoblastic leukaemia, acute myeloblastic leukaemia, Hodgkin's disease, some non-Hodgkin's lymphomas (diffuse histiocytic lymphoma, diffuse lymphoblastic lymphoma and Burkitt's lymphoma), embryonal rhabdomyosarcoma (a muscle cancer), Ewing's sarcoma (a bone cancer), Wilm's tumour (a kidney cancer), choriocarcinoma of women (cancer of the placenta), testicular cancers, ovarian cancers and a certain type of lung cancer (small cell anaplastic type). The chance of cure is much higher for some types than others. For example, it is about seven out of ten for testicular tumours overall, but only about one out of twenty for small cell lung cancer.

What happens when people with these types of cancer have chemotherapy?

First of all, for some, the outcome is complete cure. These people live as long as they would have if they had never had the cancer. Not only do they experience great benefits, the cost of their chemotherapy is partly offset by the fact that it occupies a relatively small proportion of the time between diagnosis and death.

Secondly, there are some people who are not cured but do have long complete remissions. They therefore live longer than they would have without the chemotherapy. During their remissions they are free of symptoms of cancer. If their remission is longer than their chemotherapy treatment programme, they even have some of their extra time free both of cancer symptoms and of side effects of chemotherapy.

Thirdly, others have short partial remissions. On average these people live no longer than they would have without treatment. During their short remissions they still experience some cancer symptoms as well as the side effects of their chemotherapy.

Fourthly, there are some people who do not have a remission at all. They are definitely worse off for having chemotherapy. In addition to dying of cancer just as soon as they would have anyway, they are subject to the side effects of chemotherapy during most, if not all, of their remaining time.

Finally, there are some people who actually die of tne side effects of chemotherapy. Some of these people die sooner than they would have without any treatment, some later.

The list of possible outcomes is shorter for people who have cancers that *cannot be cured* by chemotherapy. For them, the first possible outcome—cure—is not applicable.

Neither the first nor the second are applicable for the great majority of people who have chemotherapy—people who are unlikely to get a complete remission. The *best* outcome these people can hope for is the third, a partial remission—partial, temporary control of their cancer in exchange for costs which can be considerable.

There is one additional possible outcome for people who have preventive chemotherapy. Preventive chemotherapy is sometimes given as a supplement to either surgical or radiation treatment (see pages 215–18 of this chapter for a more detailed discussion of this). The aim of the chemotherapy is to prevent recurrence by eradicating any tiny seedlings which *might* still be present. Obviously the people who don't have any such seedlings—those whose cancer has actually already been cleared by the surgery or radiotherapy—cannot possibly get any benefit from the chemotherapy. They don't need it. This is another category of people for whom the cost of chemotherapy has no counterbalancing benefit.

At the beginning of this section I listed some types of cancer that *can* be cured by chemotherapy even when they are extensive. There are also some cancers where chemotherapy does result in a longer *average* length of life than occurs without chemotherapy, but no patients are cured. In other words, remissions are frequent and long enough to make a difference to the average length of life. Cancers in this category include breast cancer, non-Hodgkin's lymphomas of types other than those listed above as being curable, chronic leukaemias, multiple myeloma, and cancer of the stomach and at type of bone cancer (osteogenic sarcoma).

For most cancers, however, it is a fact that people having chemotherapy live *no longer* on average, than people not having it. Cancers in this group include those of the brain, spinal cord, skin (including melanoma), sinuses, lip, tongue, throat, larynx, oesophagus (gullet), lung (except for small cell anaplastic type), bowel, pancreas, liver, gall bladder, kidneys (except Wilm's tumour), bladder, prostate, uterus and cervix (womb and neck of womb), thyroid gland, adrenal gland, pituitary gland, bone (except for Ewing's tumour and osteogenic sarcoma) and soft tissues like muscle (except embryonal rhabdomyosarcoma in children). Given that the average length of life is no longer with treatment, it may surprise you to hear that a few people with these types of cancers do get temporary remissions. These remissions are so infrequent and short that they make no difference to the *average* length of life of people with these cancers. In spite of the fact that chemotherapy for these types of cancer does not increase the average length of life, many people with them are advised, pressured and cajoled into having chemotherapy. Think very carefully before you join their ranks.

Don't settle for overall figures when you are getting the facts together. Find out exactly what applies in your particular case. Within each cancer type, the chances depend on the exact subtype as seen under the microscope, the extent of the cancer (the site and number of deposits and the organs in which they are located) and what previous treatment has been used.

For example, the chance of curing cancer of the testis is about seven in ten overall. It is highest for a type called embryonal cell cancer (also called undifferentiated teratoma) and lowest for a type called choriocarcinoma. If the secondary cancer deposits are so small that they can neither be felt nor seen on X-rays, the chance of cure is over nine out of ten. (In these cases the presence of tiny cancer seedlings is proved by detecting certain hormones in the blood.) If secondary cancer deposits are quite small and confined to the lung or lymph glands, the chance of cure is about seven in ten. Large deposits in these sites bring the chance down to about five in ten. Any deposits in the liver reduce the chances to well under five out of ten. If they are in the brain cure is not possible. People who have already been treated unsuccessfully with chemotherapy have a much lower chance of cure than people who have not. You can see from these facts that overall figures can be very misleading for individuals. For example, it is true that the overall chance of curing testicular cancer is seven out of ten. However, it would be very misleading to tell this to a person who had already had some unsuccessful chemotherapy for choriocarcinoma of the testes in his liver. *His* particular chance would be more like one in ten.

The example I have detailed concerns only chance of cure but exactly the same sorts of differences are true for chance of remission, average length of remission, and average length of life. You must find out exactly what applies in your particular case.

COSTS OF CHEMOTHERAPY

We have just seen that many individual patients get no benefit from chemotherapy. Unfortunately, the same is not true of cost. *All* patients who have chemotherapy experience some costs, in terms of inconvenience and side effects.

A few chemotherapy drugs can be taken by mouth. Most chemotherapy drugs are given by injection, often by intravenous injection (straight into the vein). Some are given by continuous drips straight into a vein or an artery.

Some chemotherapy drugs have very few and minor side effects. However, most produce side effects which have a major impact on lifestyle and appearance. Chemotherapy often involves hospitalisation, either to actually administer the treatment or because of side effects. Some of its side effects are permanent, some are disabling, and some are dangerous. Chemotherapy, in the doses which are normally given, kills some people.

Make sure you find out what costs chemotherapy is likely to have for you by asking your doctor and reading this and the next chapter. Insist on being told the names of the proposed drugs and read about them in the next chapter. Don't make the mistake of believing that there is some sort of relationship between cost and benefit with chemotherapy.

It is very important for you to understand that severe side effects don't necessarily mean that a drug is working against a cancer. In fact, the truth is that the side effects of chemotherapy provide *no* indication as to its likely benefit. The side effects are due to damage to normal cells. The benefits come from damage to cancer cells. The two things are completely unrelated. You cannot draw any conclusions about the effect of treatment on your cancer from the severity or nature of your side effects. For example, loss of hair is neither a good sign nor a bad sign. It only means that your normal hair follicles are sensitive to the drugs you are having—nothing more. Your cancer cells may be equally or more sensitive or they may be resistant—you can't tell by what happens to your hair or by any other side effect. The effects on the *cancer* are judged by checking things to do with the cancer such as the size of known deposits, the length of remission and the length of life.

Many people believe that a treatment which makes you feel really bad must be doing some good. This is not true of chemotherapy treatment (or for any other anti-cancer treatment for that matter!)

SOME THINGS TO CONSIDER WHEN DECIDING WHETHER TO HAVE CHEMOTHERAPY

As with all decisions about treatment, you need to weigh the likely cost against the likely benefit when deciding about chemotherapy. You will have to consider all the facts you can get from your doctor about the particular treatment recommended for your particular cancer—the chance (if any) of cure, the chance of complete and of partial remission, the average length of life, the likely side effects and inconvenience of treatment. Find out what is likely to happen if you don't have the treatment or if you have any alternative treatment. In making your decision it is also essential that you take into account your own unique knowledge of yourself. You are the only one who can do that.

Try to think clearly about the most likely outcome of your treatment. I think it is especially important to compare the length of the proposed treatment programme with the average length of life. Take into account the fact that, after completing intensive chemotherapy, it often takes quite a few months to get back to feeling anything like normal.

Say you are recommended treatment that takes twelve months. The average length of life with treatment is nine months (*less* than the recommended length of treatment) and without it is six months. The chance of remission is two out of ten and cure is not possible. *With or without* this treatment, you are extremely unlikely to get any time during which you will feel completely well. If you do have this treatment, the most likely outcome is that you will simply add the inconvenience and unpleasantness of chemotherapy to the problems caused by the cancer itself, because you are not likely to get a remission. You *may* get a remission and you *may* live slightly longer if you do have the treatment, but even if you do get these so-called benefits, what will the rest of your life really be like for you? Probably worse than if you had no chemotherapy.

We are all different. The decision that is best for you might not be the one that is best for somebody else. Would you feel better if you knew you had tried every treatment with even the slightest chance of temporarily controlling your cancer? Or would you prefer to accept that the time left is short and spend it uncomplicated by the inconvenience and discomforts of chemotherapy? If your cancer is not causing a lot of discomfort at the moment, would you prefer to reserve any chemotherapy until such time as it is? If it is causing problems, are there other ways of treating the symptoms besides trying to control the cancer itself?

Even if you have found out all the facts about your cancer and the proposed treatment, your decision will still have to be based on what is *likely* to happen rather than what will *definitely* happen. As we have already discussed, no one can look into the future and see exactly what will happen to you as an individual. They *can* tell you what is likely, what is possible and what is very unlikely. You must base your initial decision on this. Don't forget you can always revise your decision later in the light of what actually does happen to you. It might help to re-read pages 93–95 here.

I know that some of you will decide to have chemotherapy even when you know the chances of it lengthening your life or improving its quality are very small. That's up to you. You know what you want.

The important thing is not the decision you make, but the fact that it is based on a realistic understanding of your situation. If it is, you will be in control of the situation. Your expectations will be realistic. You will be in a position to evaluate what actually happens to you and then to make further decisions in your own best interests as time goes by.

Never decide to have chemotherapy treatment before discussing it with a doctor who is experienced in its use. Make sure your doses are calculated and the treatment supervised overall by an experienced chemotherapy doctor. Chemotherapy is dangerous. Doses which can control cancer have serious side effects. Doses which are normally used can and do kill some people.

You will need an expert who knows how the drugs work, what types of cancer they are likely to act against, and how to calculate doses that are reasonably safe while still having a chance of being effective against your cancer. But don't forget all the warnings I have given you about experts. You need their expertise and specialised knowledge but don't rely on them to make the best judgements and decisions on your behalf.

It is likely that it will be hard work getting all the information you need to make your own decisions—be prepared for this. Unless you have a type of cancer which is very sensitive to chemotherapy, your doctors will probably be very reluctant to explain just what outcomes chemotherapy is likely to have for you. The reasons are obvious. Firstly, your doctors might look and feel rather foolish trying to explain just why they want you to have treatment that is likely to make you feel quite unwell but very unlikely to result in you living any longer. Secondly, if they did explain all this they would be risking losing control of the situation—you might refuse to accept their recommendations.

What some doctors try to do is give no information, just orders. Others may *appear* to be willing to share information—they may explain in detail about the costs of chemotherapy but omit to explain exactly what the likely benefits are. They know by experience that the best way to ensure that people do take their advice is to leave a lot unsaid. They know that people will then make assumptions about the situation along these sorts of lines: 'The treatment sounds so nasty that it *must* do a lot of good. I was hoping against hope that they would be able to do something for me and now it looks as though they can. No one would recommend such unpleasant, inconvenient and dangerous treatment unless there was a high chance that it would control the cancer for a long time, maybe even cure me.' Unfortunately the conclusions reached by this hopeful, sensible and logical sort of reasoning are often very wrong. The fact is, chemotherapy is often recommended when there is no chance of cure. It is often recommended when there is only a small chance of a short remission. It is often recommended when it makes no difference to the average length of life.

So, don't guess. Don't assume that recommendations are based on commonsense. Don't let your need to maintain hope prevent you from facing the facts. *Never agree to chemotherapy without knowing both sides of the cost/benefit balance.*

People who do agree to treatment without knowing all the

important facts often enter a vicious circle where they make similar decisions repeatedly. Say, for example, that on the basis of the sort of reasoning I have outlined, a person agrees to have chemotherapy that is actually very unlikely to produce a remission. Two months later the doctor says: 'I'm afraid your treatment isn't working. I recommend you try some different chemotherapy drugs.' The fact that the treatment isn't working is no surprise to the doctor, but it is to the patient who then assumes that he or she has just been very unlucky. After all, how can they possibly know *now* that what has happened to them is not exceptional, but typical, if they didn't know to *start* with that their treatment was unlikely to produce a remission? They think: 'I can't be so unlucky twice. I'll try the new treatment.' And so the cycle repeats, often more than once. Make sure that *you* don't fall into this sort of pattern by making sure that *you* decide what to do on the basis of facts, not assumptions.

I've explained *how* some doctors persuade their patients to have treatment which carries very much greater cost than benefit. But *why* do doctors do this. What can possibly motivate them?

They would probably say things like: 'While there's life, there's hope' or 'It would be cruel not to try every treatment that could possibly control the cancer'. The real reasons, in my opinion, are to do with the doctors' need to look and feel powerful. We discussed this to some extent in Chapter 5. These doctors have decided to make a career of fighting cancer. Their top priority is to defeat the cancer itself, not to care for the whole person with cancer. These doctors find it very difficult to face up to the real situation when they have a patient whose cancer is very unlikely to be controlled by any form of treatment. They are not prepared to admit this to themselves or their patient. They avoid admitting it by recommending further treatment — any treatment which has any chance at all of temporarily having some effect on the cancer. This treatment is often chemotherapy — either in a form that is definitely very unlikely to produce a temporary remission or some variation on such treatment, that just might be better.

Here is an example of what I mean. The 'best' drug for secondary colon cancer is called fluorouracil. Although this drug is reasonably active against some other types of cancer, with colon cancer it produces only occasional short remissions and makes no difference to the average length of life. Yet thousands and thousands of patients with colon cancer have been given fluorouracil. They have been given it by mouth, by intravenous injection, by intravenous drip, and by a drip straight into the artery that goes to the liver. They have been given it in single large doses, weekly small doses, intensive courses followed by weekly injections and continuous drips over months. They have been given it combined with a great number of other drugs. They have been given it as a supplement to complete surgical removal of primary bowel cancer in an effort to prevent secondary cancer forming. They have been given various closely related chemicals. And still, there is no evidence that it ever makes any difference to the average length of life. Every one of these thousands and thousands of patients has experienced inconvenience and discomfort in order for doctors to confirm over and over again that fluoroucil has very little effect on colon cancer.

Yet many patients are still advised to have this treatment! *You* must decide whether *you* want to be a part of such never ending quests.

Don't think this is an isolated example. It's not – the same sort of thing happens with every type of cancer that is rarely responsive to chemotherapy. If you have one of these types, consider especially carefully what you, as an individual, are likely to gain or to lose by having chemotherapy.

WHY CHEMOTHERAPY CAN'T CURE ALL CANCER

In spite of the fact that chemotherapy travels throughout the body and so can get to nearly every cancer cell, we have seen that many types of cancer cannot by cured by chemotherapy. Why not?

The reason is quite simple.

Most cells of most types of cancer are *less* sensitive to the damaging effects of chemotherapy than many normal cells. Doses of chemotherapy drugs which are so high that they regularly produce very unpleasant and dangerous side effects (because of extensive damage to normal cells) are still not high enough to destroy most types of cancer cells. It's simply impossible to give enough chemotherapy to cure most types of cancer because the required dose would kill the person with the cancer first.

Attempts have been made to improve chemotherapy. Approaches include searching for new drugs and testing new ways of using the currently available ones.

WAYS OF TRYING TO IMPROVE THE BENEFITS OF CHEMOTHERAPY

Most people doing research on cancer treatment concentrate on trying to improve benefits rather than on trying to reduce costs.

Their usual aim is to develop treatments which can produce more frequent or longer remissions. Some research on reducing side effects is done, but not usually with the primary aim of making treatment more pleasant for people. The primary aim is usually to allow doctors to give more of the drug. The side effects which get research attention are those which limit what the 'experts' can do—for example, those that are frequently fatal or so severe that people refuse to continue with their treatment.

For example, nausea and vomiting are side effects of many chemotherapy drugs. Little attention was given to this problem until a drug called cis-platinum came into use. Cis-platinum produced such frequent and severe nausea and vomiting that even some patients who had a good chance of cure refused to continue treatment with it. This was the lever needed—a great deal of research has since gone into ways of reducing or controlling the nausea and vomiting produced by chemotherapy drugs.

New Drugs

As I have mentioned, most currently available chemotherapy drugs do as much, or more, damage to some of our normal cells as they do to cancer cells. The reactions of the normal tissues make it impossible to give these drugs in high enough doses, often enough, to kill all the cancer cells. Therefore a lot of effort is put into finding or developing new drugs which will do more damage to cancer cells than to normal cells. Some of this research is done on a logical basis, for example, various close relatives of currently available drugs are developed for testing in case one of them proves to be better than the one already in use. Thousands of naturally occurring and synthetic chemical compounds are also screened in the laboratory for any indication that they could be harmful to cancer cells. So far, it is a fact that most of the drugs actually in use have been found by luck or screening, rather than by any logical process. Re-read pages 95–96 if you want to refresh your memory about the different phases of testing drugs in humans, once they have shown some promise in laboratory testing. It would be especially important to re-read this section if you have been asked to take part in research on new drugs.

Use Of Multiple Drugs

Nowadays, chemotherapy drugs are rarely used singly. Usually, two, three or more drugs are given at the same time. The reason for this is that combining drugs is a relatively safe way of increasing the damage done to the cancer cells. Giving three times the maximum safe dose of a single drug is not a practical way of trebling the damage done to the cancer cells. The risk of killing the patient would be much too high. However, the damage to the cancer cells *can* be trebled fairly safely by giving three *different* drugs at the same time, each in its maximum safe dose.

Here is an example. Cis-platinum, bleomycin and vinblastine are three drugs that are active against testicular cancer. While each of these drugs used on its own can produce temporary remissions, they rarely produce cures. The normal tissue that is most sensitive to cis-platinum is the kidney. The normal tissue whose reaction limits the dose to bleomycin is the lung. The normal tissues which are most sensitive to vinblastine are the bone marrow and the nerves. In other words, the safe dose of each drug is determined by the reactions of different tissues. This makes it possible to give a safe maximum dose of all three drugs at the same time. And in fact this combination has been used very successfully—it will cure more than seven out of ten people with extensive testicular cancer. Unfortunately, it is nowhere near as effective against any other type of cancer, with one exception—a rare type of cancer of the ovary which is the female counterpart of the testicular cancer. The common type of cancer of the ovary is nowhere near as sensitive to this drug combination.

This particular example is one of a small number of drug combinations which definitely produce much greater benefits than single drugs. There are a few other types of cancer for which combinations that greatly improve the cure rate have been developed. These include Hodgkin's disease, acute lymphoblastic leukaemia of children, rhabdomyosarcoma, and Ewing's sarcoma. However, as you know, most types of cancer can never be cured by chemotherapy, whether drugs are used singly or in combination. For most types of cancer, the advantages of combination treatment are either less dramatic or even non-existent.

There are some types of cancer where combinations of drugs do definitely produce a higher remission rate, longer average remissions and longer average length of life, although they produce no cures. Secondary breast cancer is one of these. In this type of cancer, the highest remission rate which can be achieved with a single drug is about one in three. When multiple drugs are used the remission rate can be about two in three, more of the remissions are complete (no *detectable* cancer remaining) and the remissions last longer. These people also live longer, on average, but chemotherapy never *cures* people with secondary breast cancer.

Unfortunately, many drug combinations produce results that are no better than when drugs are used on their own. To take an extreme case, drugs that are useless against a particular type of cancer on their own are still useless when used in combination. For example, for the most common type of lung cancer (squamous cell cancer), there is no drug or combination of drugs which have been shown to result in people living longer, on average, than they do with no treatment. Some drugs can produce short remissions in a small proportion of patients but when combined they still produce only short remissions in a small proportion of patients. Very few remissions are complete and very few remissions last more than a few months. Drug combinations do not *necessarily* produce better results than single drugs.

The one fact about combination treatments that can be stated with complete certainty is that they *always* produce more inconvenience and discomfort than single drugs and much, much more inconvenience and discomfort than no treatment at all. That means they are not worth having unless there are some definite benefits to counterbalance these costs.

If you are advised to have a combination of drugs, try to find out what its advantages and disadvantages are. Can it cure your type of cancer? What is the chance of remission? What is the average length of remission? What is the average length of life? How does this compare with the situation if you had only one drug? Or no drugs? You need all this information before you decide whether or not to accept a drug combination.

Adjuvant Chemotherapy

The word 'adjuvant' means helpful or auxiliary. Adjuvant chemotherapy is chemotherapy given in addition to either surgical removal or radiation treatment of all *known* cancer deposits. It is chemotherapy added to a treatment which actually does cure some people on its own. The idea of adding the chemotherapy is to improve the cure rate, or, failing that, to at least increase the average length of remission and average length of life.

For all types of cancer the best chance of complete cure is at the time when localised cancer is first diagnosed. In fact, for most types of cancer this is the *only* time when there is any chance of a complete cure. As we now know, most cancers cannot be cured once obvious secondary growths have formed. Adjuvant chemotherapy was devised in an attempt to solve this problem. By giving chemotherapy *before* any tiny seedlings left after local treatment had a chance to grow, maybe we could completely

215

prevent, or at least delay, the formation of obvious secondary growths.

That's the theory. What are the results of applying it? There are some types of cancer where the average length of remission and average length of life are indeed definitely increased by the use of adjuvant chemotherapy. They include cancer of the muscle in children (rhabdomyosarcoma), a type of kidney cancer (Wilm's tumour), some bone cancers (Ewing's sarcoma and osteogenic sarcoma), Burkitt's lymphoma, localised diffuse histiocytic lymphoma, small cell anaplastic cancer of the lung and stage two breast cancer (cancer which has spread to the lymph nodes in the armpit). In the case of breast cancer, an improved average length of remission and of life are definite only for women who are still menstruating and who only had one or two nodes affected by their cancer. It is almost certain that the addition of adjuvant chemotherapy increases the rate of complete and permanent cure of all of these cancers with the exception of breast cancer. The eventual cure rate of breast cancer is at best improved by less than ten per cent (one in ten) and may not be improved at all.

I cannot be completely definite about the impact of adjuvant chemotherapy on cure rates because it has not been in use for long enough, and it is known to change the timing of recurrence in some types of cancer. For example, if a person with osteogenic sarcoma is treated *only* by surgery and has no recurrence within the next two years, we can be almost completely sure that they have been cured. *Without* adjuvant chemotherapy, this type of cancer practically always recurs within two years if it is going to recur at all. Adjuvant chemotherapy changes that pattern. Some people who have had adjuvant chemotherapy for osteogenic sarcoma have had recurrence five or more years after diagnosis. These people certainly had their remissions greatly extended but were not cured. If we follow them up for long enough we could even find that eventually no extra people are cured of osteogenic sarcoma by adjuvant chemotherapy. It is possible that as many people will eventually relapse as would have anyway without adjuvant chemotherapy, although so far this has not happened. We need much longer follow-ups to be absolutely certain of cures, because adjuvant chemotherapy changes the pattern of recurrence.

Late recurrences are also known to occur with Ewing's sarcoma and Burkitt's lymphoma. However, with rhabdomyosarcoma and diffuse histiocytic lymphoma, for example, they don't seem to happen—any recurrences that are going to occur usually do so during chemotherapy or within a few months of stopping it. We can be much more confident that we *are* getting extra cures with these cancers.

Of course, this doubt about the eventual cure rate doesn't mean that adjuvant chemotherapy has no definite benefits. In the cancers I listed it does definitely extend the average length of remission and length of life, sometimes by many years.

Unfortunately, cancers where adjuvant chemotherapy does make a difference are the exceptions. For most types of cancer, adjuvant chemotherapy makes no difference to the average length of remission, length of life or cure rate. On page 204 of this chapter there is a list of cancers where chemotherapy does no more than produce occasional short remissions when it is used against secondary cancer. Using chemotherapy before secondary cancer is evident does not improve the outlook for these types of cancer. Their cells are simply not very sensitive to any currently available drugs. Using the same drugs when there are only a few cells present (adjuvant chemotherapy) doesn't alter that fact.

For those of you who are seriously considering having adjuvant chemotherapy because you have a type of cancer whose outcome is favourably influenced by it, there is one more fact that you should take into account. You, as an individual, may not need any additional treatment, because you may not have any cancer cells left. They may already have been cleared by your surgery or radiation.

The only people who can possibly benefit from adjuvant chemotherapy are those who *do* have some cells left. And only some of these people benefit—the ones whose cells are sensitive to the drugs. Unfortunately, there is no way of definitely telling whether or not you are one of these people beforehand. You must make your decision on the basis of chances.

If you ask your doctor directly what your chance is of still having any cancer cells after local treatment, you will probably get an evasive answer. You can get the answer indirectly by asking your doctor what your chance of recurrence would be if you *didn't* have chemotherapy. The chance that there are still cells in your body after the local treatment is exactly the same, because it is these cells that would give rise to any recurrence. For example, if your chance of recurrence *without* adjuvant chemotherapy is seventy per cent, there is a seven in ten chance that you still have cancer cells in your body and a three in ten chance that you do not.

To find out the chance of any remaining cells being sensitive to the proposed chemotherapy, ask what the chance of remission is when the same drugs are given to a person with secondary cancer. Any cells that you still have have about the same chance of being sensitive to the treatment. If only occasional remissions can be produced in secondary cancer of your type, adjuvant chemotherapy is very unlikely to help you.

Find out what your situation would be if you don't have the adjuvant chemotherapy now, but just wait and see whether you are one of the unlucky ones who does get a recurrence. What chance of cure, if any, would there be at that stage? What chance of remission? What is the average length of remission? What is the average length of life? Compare this to the chance of cure, average length of remission and average length of life with adjuvant chemotherapy. Take into consideration the length of the chemotherapy programme.

Your decision should be influenced by your personal preferences. Don't be apologetic or embarrassed about considering them— they're important. Would you prefer to take every treatment that could possibly make you live longer? Or would you prefer to take your chances and about having chemotherapy if, and when, your cancer recurs? Are the side effects of treatment things that you would find extremely hard or relatively easy to cope with? *You* decide what's best for you.

Treatment Programmes

Another way of trying to get more out of the available chemotherapy drugs is by experimenting with variations in treatment programmes—different drug combinations, sequences, dosage, and timing. A great deal of research effort goes into this sort of testing. Some variations are based on theories. Some are based on the results of previous research in test tubes, animals or other people. Some are purely determined by what is possible—pushing to the limits the number of drugs, their dosage and how often they are given. The variations are rarely designed to reduce inconvenience or side effects, unless these are so severe that too many people refuse the treatment or die as a result of it.

It is a fact that changing the dose, sequence and timing of some treatments can change the results. For example, most chemotherapy treatment is given over a few days in high doses with two or three week recovery periods between treatments. This sort of programme has been found to have a much better chance of controlling most types of cancer than when low doses of the same drugs are given every day. However, the high dose intermittent treatment also has more side effects. This brings me to a general rule—any variation in treatment that produces a greater effect on the cancer usually does so at a greater cost. The reverse is not true, many variations which increase the cost make no difference to the benefits. Especially when the drugs being used have little effect against the particular cancer under study, variations often produce greater side effects and inconvenience without any added benefit. You need only look back at what I have said about the use of fluorouracil in colon cancer (pages 210–11) to confirm this.

When your proposed treatment programme is described to you, you may be surprised at how inconvenient and complicated it sounds. It is sometimes worth questioning this. Often there is no real evidence that a complicated and inconvenient programme is any better than a much simpler one. Why would your doctors recommend it then? Well, unless they are doing research themselves, the recommended treatment will be the one they have decided is the 'best'. Re-read pages 88–93 if you want to remind yourself about how doctors decide which treatment is 'best'. Remember, it is usually the one that is reported to have the highest remission rate, and longest average length of life, almost regardless of any consideration of cost. Your doctors will read medical books and journals, decide on the 'best' treatment and then recommend that you have exactly that treatment, given in exactly the same way. They will be reluctant to alter any detail of how it is given, because scientifically trained doctors are taught to give the exact treatment that is scientifically shown to be the 'best'.

So, for example, if the 'best' treatment includes cis-platinum given in small doses intravenously for five days running every three weeks, that's what will be recommended, even though your doctor should know that if the entire dose is given on one day you get the same benefits but a shorter period of inconvenience and nausea. If it includes fluorouracil given by a continuous drip, that's what will be recommended, even though your doctor should know that this works no better than giving it as a rapid intravenous injection. If it includes drugs given direct into the artery, that's what will be recommended, even though your doctor should know that there is no evidence that *any* drugs work better when given this way than when given into the vein.

So it is worth querying any aspect of your treatment that seems particularly inconvenient or unpleasant. Ask whether the drugs can be given any other way. Ask what the results would be with more simple treatment. Ask just what *extra* benefit, if any, is likely to result from the proposed programme. Beware of explanations that rely completely on theory. You don't want to know whether it is likely in theory that this programme will get better results — you want to know what results it actually produces. If they can't tell you what results it actually produces, they are really recommending a research treatment, whatever they may call it. You should recognise that in deciding whether or not to accept it. Re-read pages 95–100 if a research treatment is recommended for you.

Length of Treatment Programme

One aspect of treatment programmes that I'd like to discuss more fully is the total length of the programme. Many patients are advised to continue chemotherapy for long periods of time when it is very unlikely that they will gain any additional benefit from doing so. Obviously, the longer treatment goes on for, the more it 'costs'. How can you tell when there is unlikely to be any further benefit from continuing your treatment? What you must insist on being told is what is happening to the *size of your cancer deposits*.

If your cancer is bigger than when you started the treatment, its cells are not sensitive to those particular drugs. There is *never* anything to be gained by continuing the same treatment in this situation.

If your cancer has not changed in size after a few months of treatment, you stand to gain very little, if anything, from continuing chemotherapy. You are just adding the inconvenience and side effects of chemotherapy to your cancer symptoms (which won't have improved if the cancer is no smaller). This chemotherapy is unlikely to extend your life and certainly will never produce a complete remission or cure.

If your cancer is smaller, its cells are definitely being destroyed by the treatment. There is some benefit to be gained by continuing this treatment. It will probably make the cancer smaller still, or even produce a complete remission (no detectable cancer left).

What about when a complete remission is reached? For how much longer is continuing treatment likely to bring additional benefit? The first thing I'll remind you of is that a complete remission doesn't mean there is definitely no cancer left in your body. It means only that there are no cancer deposits bigger than about 1cm across—that is, big enough to feel, or see on an X-ray or scan. Once there is no longer any detectable cancer, there is no longer any guide as to whether or not continuing treatment is causing further reduction in the numbers of cells. We certainly can't tell for sure when, if ever, there are no cancer cells left.

There are a few special types of cancer where we can tell exactly what's happening even when there are extremely small numbers of cells left. These are choriocarcinoma of women and some cancers of the testis (including choriocarcinoma of men). These cancers release into the bloodstream a particular hormone which can be accurately measured. It has been found that the chance of cure and the average length of life are not improved by continuing treatment for any more than six or eight weeks after such time as these hormones become either undetectable or reach normal levels.

How long should treatment go on after a complete remission is reached in all the types of cancer which don't have these useful hormone markers? Many doctors recommend that treatment continue for many months or even years. When they have no way of knowing for sure whether there is any cancer left, they prefer to risk over-treatment rather than under-treatment. That would be fine if there was no cost attached to such over-treatment, but of course there is and you're the one who would pay it.

I believe that it is extremely unlikely that the chance of cure, if any, and average length of life are improved by continuing treatment for more than a few months, six at the very most, after 'complete' remission is diagnosed. However, continuing treatment may make the remission last longer. This doesn't result in a longer average life span, because when people continue treatment throughout a remission, it is very hard to get a second remission when they do relapse. People who stop treatment during a remission are much easier to get into a second remission when they relapse. Although they tend to relapse sooner (but not more often), the fact that they then have a better chance of responding to re-treatment means that their eventual length of life is about the same.

You must decide which scenario you prefer if your doctor recommends continuing treatment long after you enter a complete remission. Obviously your decision would be influenced by the cost of your particular treatment. Some cancers which can only be brought into remission with intensive treatment can be kept in remission with much milder treatment. An example is acute leukaemia.

If you are having preventive treatment, you and your doctor can't use the size of your cancer as a guide to treatment because you don't have any detectable cancer. You will have to be guided by the length of treatment that has been successful with other people.

Basically, I want you to realise that your responsibility to yourself doesn't end with deciding to start a treatment. You need to keep weighing the cost against the benefit *during* the treatment. You should stop your treatment whenever, for you, the cost is greater than the benefit. Provided you can get the required information, you are the best person to decide when that time has come.

Artificial Feeding

Many people believe that, if only they could fatten themselves up, things would somehow be better. A lot of doctors also believe in trying to 'fatten up' people who are either having chemotherapy or for whom it is planned. Does artificial feeding, given either intravenously or through a tube going via the nose into the stomach, actually improve the results of chemotherapy?

These are the facts. Firstly, a well-nourished person does tend to live longer. Secondly, a well-nourished person tends to have less side effects from chemotherapy than a poorly-nourished one. That's all. A well-nourished person is no more likely to get a remission or to be cured. The cancer cells of a well-nourished person are not more likely than those of a poorly-nourished person to be sensitive to chemotherapy.

If you are considering artificial feeding, you need to find out what, if anything, you stand to gain from it and at what cost. Personally, I would only ever agree to it myself if I was so undernourished that I was not fit to take intensive chemotherapy which had a *high* chance of *curing* me. I think in all other cases the benefits are too slight to justify the costs. However, you must weigh the cost/benefit balance for yourself.

Artificial feeding might result in you having less side effects from chemotherapy, but would the extra cost of the artificial feeding outweigh the benefit for you? You might gain a greater length of life, but how is that extra life likely to be for you? The chance of the cancer going into remission is no better. If it does go into remission, your general health will improve anyway. If it doesn't go into remission, any extra time will probably be unpleasant. Your cancer will have extra time to grow and give rise to new symptoms. On top of that you will have to cope with the inconvenience and discomfort of the artificial feeding and any chemotherapy treatment you have. Perhaps, for you, any extension of life is worthwhile regardless of the direct and indirect costs. If not, I suggest you consider the situation very carefully before you agree to artificial feeding.

Protection From Infection

Infections are a common cause of death in people with cancer, especially people who are having chemotherapy. This fact has prompted doctors to investigate the possibility that the results of chemotherapy would be improved if infection could be prevented. The procedures necessary to significantly reduce the risk of infection are so costly, inconvenient and depersonalising, and the benefits so minor, that I would never agree to them for myself. However, I will describe them for you so you can make up your own mind.

To reduce your chance of infection, you would have to be cleared of the germs that are normally in and on your body and then isolated from any other germs. The germs normally in and on you would be reduced by washing regularly with antiseptic, putting antiseptic or antibiotics in your nose, eyes, ears and vagina, using antiseptic mouth washes and taking antibiotics to kill the germs that are normally in your bowels. You could be protected from outside germs by being isolated in a special enclosed unit which is ventilated with sterilised air. Nothing that was not first sterilised would be allowed in your room. You could not touch another person. The need for anyone to come into your room would be minimised by doing as much as possible from

224

outside, using plastic sleeves that project into the room. If anyone did have to come in they would be completely covered from head to foot with a sterile cap, mask, gown, gloves and boots.

What are the benefits of these cumbersome procedures? Well, people with leukaemia and other forms of cancer who are treated like this do have fewer days with infection than people who are not. But that's all — their average length of life, chance of remission and chance of cure is no different. Protecting people from infection doesn't make their cancer cells any more sensitive to chemotherapy — it just reduces their chance of infection. If this sort of protective nursing is recommended for you, you must decide whether the only definite benefit — fewer days with infection — justifies the cost.

Bone Marrow Transplantation

Damage to the bone marrow is the side effect that limits the dose of many chemotherapy drugs. One way of trying to overcome this limitation is with bone marrow transplantation. This is a procedure I would never agree to for myself. To help you form your own opinion if it has been recommended for you, here's a brief description of what it would involve.

First, you would undergo the procedures to reduce the chances of infection that I described in the last section. Next, you would be given such huge doses of radiotherapy and chemotherapy that all of your own bone marrow cells would definitely be permanently destroyed. Ideally, but by no means definitely, this extremely intensive treatment would also destroy all your cancer cells. New bone marrow would then be injected into your blood, hopefully to give rise to new blood-forming marrow in your bones over the next few months. Until this happens, you would have to remain in your sterile isolation unit.

The results? Well, this sort of treatment *can* cure cancer but *only if* the transplant is not rejected *and if* the transplanted marrow cells don't attack the recipient's own cells *and if* all the cancer cells are indeed destroyed *and if* the chemotherapy and radiotherapy don't cause fatal damage to some other part of the body.

The only type of cancer which has more than a minute chance of being cured by this very costly, inconvenient and unpleasant treatment is leukaemia. The chance depends on the exact type and stage of the leukaemia and what treatment the person has previously had. If bone marrow transplantation is recommended for you, try to find out exactly what it will involve and what your own chances really are— of temporary remission and of cure. The costs are very high, so you would need to be sure that the likely benefit was also very high before agreeing to it.

Sanctuary Sites

I mentioned right at the beginning of this chapter that most chemotherapy drugs do not penetrate properly into the central nervous system (brain, spinal cord and cerebro-spinal fluid), ovaries and testes. These are called **sanctuary sites** because any cancer cells which lodge there have effectively found a fairly safe and protected hiding place from chemotherapy.

The central nervous system is a much more common site for secondary deposits than the ovaries and testes, so this is the area that most often needs to be tackled in special ways. Radiation is one means of doing this. There are also certain chemotherapy drugs which do penetrate into the central nervous system— they include methotretate when given in very high doses, nitrosoureas, procarbazine and cytosine arabinoside.

A third method— injecting chemotherapy drugs into the cerebro-spinal fluid— is only useful when the cancer cells are confined to this fluid and not in the brain itself. The cerebro-spinal fluid surrounds the brain and spinal cord and also flows through special channels inside the brain. One way of getting drugs into the cerebro-spinal fluid is through an injection near the base of the spine— the same as a lumbar puncture (see pages 79–80). If you dislike lumbar punctures and would want to have repeated injections into the cerebro-spinal fluid, an alternative is to have them given through an Ommaya-type reservoir. This is a special device that makes it very easy to give injections directly into the cerebro-spinal fluid in the brain. An operation is necessary to put it in place. Under anaesthetic, a small circle of skull bone is removed. One end of a fine pointed hollow tube is then pushed through the brain into one of the internal cerebro-spinal fluid channels. Its position is checked with X-rays. The other lies just under the skin of the skull. Injections made through the skin into this tube will go straight into the cerebro-spinal fluid. Once the Ommaya-type reservoir is in place, it is very easy to give these injections and to get samples of cerebro-spinal fluid for testing.

Before deciding on any treatment for cancer in the brain or cerebro-spinal fluid it is important that you realise that there is *no* type of cancer that can be cured once it has definitely spread into the central nervous system. If you have a cancer which has done this, I suggest you consider your position very carefully before agreeing to any treatment. Cure isn't possible. Complete control of your symptoms is very unlikely. Any extra time you might gain is likely to be short and occupied by rather inconvenient treatment. You will probably still die in the same way as you would without the treatment, but maybe a bit later. It's grim and, as is so often the case with cancer, there are no nice alternatives. You have to choose the least unpleasant of the alternatives there are.

These sorts of treatments are not recommended only for treating definite secondary cancer in the central nervous system. They are also sometimes recommended in an attempt to *prevent* it from developing. It's similar to the situation with adjuvant chemotherapy treatment for cancer that *might* be there. If this is recommended, find out just what the proposed treatment would involve. How likely is central nervous system cancer to develop if you have this treatment? And if you don't? If you could be cured, would this treatment improve your chance of cure? By how much? What side effects could you have both at the time of the treatment and later on? These are the sorts of questions you need answers to before agreeing to such treatment.

Getting Into Veins

Many chemotherapy drugs are given by intravenous injection. This means through a needle stuck into a vein—in the same way as blood specimens are taken, except that something is being put in rather than taken out. Before they even have any chemo-

227

therapy, some people have small veins that are hard to get needles into. However they start off, most people having chemotherapy finish up with veins that are hard to get needles into. Why does this happen? Firstly, just sticking needles into veins causes some scarring. Secondly, many chemotherapy drugs are very irritating to the lining of the vein. They cause a reaction which thickens the lining and makes it much harder to get the needle into the right spot. Intravenous drips and some antibiotics can also do this. For some people, the actual process of getting the needle into the vein becomes the most dreaded and unpleasant part of their treatment.

There are ways of getting around this. Firstly, the problem can be minimised if the finest needle that will do the job is used. Secondly, if you are having chemotherapy, do all you can to avoid having inexperienced people poking around at your veins. They are too precious for that. Next, ask whether there is any other way of giving your drugs. Some can be taken by mouth and some can be given by injection under the skin (subcutaneous) or into the muscle (intra-muscular)—check them in the next chapter. You can make your veins enlarge a bit by exercising your arm and making sure you are warm. Being relaxed also helps, although I know this is much easier said than done!

If you dread having intravenous treatment, either because your veins are difficult or simply because you hate needles, ask about having one of the following procedures done. A small operation can be done to connect an artery to a vein in the forearm (the technical name for this is an arterio-venous fistula). This increases the pressure in that vein so that over about six weeks the veins below it enlarge. Your injections will still have to go through the skin but should be much easier.

Another possibility is to have a special long, fine plastic tube placed into one of the very large veins in the lower neck. These are called Hickman's catheters. They are inserted under general or local anaesthetic and the tube is threaded under the skin to come out somewhere on the chest wall well away from your vein. Discuss with the surgeon beforehand just where you would like this to be. The reason for threading it under the skin is to reduce the risk of any infection getting into the blood. Blood can be taken from, and injections given into, the end of the catheter. It can also be used for intravenous drips. These catheters can be left in place for several years if necessary, but do require quite a bit of care. The spot where the catheter comes through the skin has to be carefully cleaned with antiseptic every day. In addition, a small amount of heparin (a drug which stops blood clotting) must be put into the tube at intervals to prevent it from blocking up. There is a definite risk of infection with these catheters. If they do get infected, they often have to be removed. A new one can be inserted to replace the infected one.

Don't wait for your doctor to recommend one of these procedures. Some doctors will wait until it's almost impossible to get a needle into a vein. You can ask about it whenever you feel that the benefits are likely to outweigh the costs for you.

Well, that covers all of the important general things you need to understand about chemotherapy. In the next chapter we will discuss the details of the individual drugs and their side effects.

CHEMOTHERAPY –
THE INDIVIDUAL DRUGS
AND THEIR SIDE EFFECTS

Chapter 10

In the first part of this chapter I will describe the side effects which are common to many chemotherapy drugs. I will then tell you about each individual drug listing their side effects and describing the ones which have not been covered in the first part of the chapter.

You will find the drugs listed in alphabetical order under a chemical name that is recognised worldwide. In different countries these drugs have different proprietary names (names given to them by the manufacturer). If you can't find one of your drugs on this list, it could be because you have been given the proprietary name. Ask your doctor what other names the drug has or ask him or her to identify it in this chapter. Alternatively, it may be a hormone rather than a chemotherapy drug, in which case you will need to check the next chapter. The third possibility is that it is a drug that is used rarely or which was still in the research stage at the time of writing this book. In that case, I hope the general information in this book will help you to work out what questions to ask your doctor and how to make sense of his or her answers.

When reading about the possible side effects of your proposed treatment, keep in mind that not all of them would happen to you. Remember that not even the common ones happen to every person who has the drug. Hardly anybody gets either every possible side effect or none at all. Most people are somewhere in between, so *you* are likely to be somewhere in between.

The doses for your first course of treatment should be worked out on the basis of your age, size, blood counts, liver and kidney function and type and extent of cancer. For later courses those doses should be adjusted according to your individual reaction.

In working out dose adjustments, your doctors should consider both your symptoms and the results of blood tests. They can't do this unless you tell them exactly what side effects you experienced and how much they worried you. Some doctors will discourage you from telling them about side effects and will be reluctant to change your doses because of them. They think that as long as you got through the side effects once, you can get through them again and again. *You* have to decide whether the possible benefit justifies the cost. If you decide it doesn't, you must tell your doctor very clearly that the costs must be reduced. Find out how the particular side effects which distressed you can be prevented or treated. Perhaps the side effect could be treated more effectively when it develops. It can always be prevented, but often prevention means reducing the dose of one or more of your chemotherapy drugs, cutting one or more out or even stopping chemotherapy altogether. These steps will of course reduce the possible benefit, but that doesn't mean they shouldn't be taken. The possible benefit may be too small to justify the cost. You decide what is best for you.

Your doctors may tell you that you are weak, lacking in determination, selfish and inconsiderate of family and friends if you insist on refusing, modifying or stopping treatment. Try not to let such accusations deter you. The doctors make them because they don't like anyone to flout their authority. You and I know that it takes a strong and courageous person to weigh up a situation and make their own decisions. You and I know that this is not taking the easy way out—doing what is best *for you* can be very hard.

GENERAL SIDE EFFECTS OF CHEMOTHERAPY

Hair Loss (Alopecia)

Chemotherapy drugs can cause temporary loss of hair by damaging the cells of the hair follicles. The hair loss can occur gradually over some weeks or suddenly over a day or two. The sudden type of loss, if it is going to happen at all, is usually within the first two weeks of treatment. The most sensitive hair is the most rapidly growing hair and that is the hair on your head. The least sensitive hair is hair that normally stays the same length, that is, hair of eyebrows, eyelashes, armpits, pubic area and general body hair. This stable hair is affected by only a few chemotherapy drugs, for example, adriamycin. If you haven't lost your hair within two months of starting treatment, you probably won't lose it with the particular drugs you are having. Of course, you still could with different ones.

The hair loss is never permanent. You can be sure that it will grow back within a few months of stopping your chemotherapy. In some cases it even starts to grow before chemotherapy is finished—the hair follicles can develop a resistance to the drugs. The new hair may initially be darker in colour, finer and curlier than the original hair. However, over some years it usually finishes up looking like the original hair. Unfortunately, this new hair is likely to fall out again whenever you start on different chemotherapy drugs or start back on the original ones after a break.

Until your hair grows again you may like to keep your head covered with a wig, scarf or hat. If you live in a country with a national health system or have medical insurance, you may be able to get a free wig. Ask your doctor what financial help is available. If you can afford it, get a good wig and have it fitted *before* you lose your hair. You can then match the colour and style more easily and will be prepared when and if you hair starts to fall out.

Several ways of trying to reduce hair loss have been tried, with very little success. These methods involve reducing the blood supply to the scalp while the drug is actually being injected. This can be done either with a very tight band around the head or by cooling the scalp. The methods are only suitable for treatment that is given entirely by rapid intravenous injections, because the band or cold pack cannot be kept in place for long periods of time. Even if they are given by rapid intravenous injection, most drugs remain in the blood much longer than the twenty or thirty minutes that a band or cold pack cap can be left in place without severe discomfort or risk of damage to the scalp. Thus it is not really surprising that these methods make very little difference to the risk of hair loss.

Damage To Bone Marrow Cells—Reduced Blood Counts

New red blood cells, platelets and most types of white blood cells are normally released continuously from the bone marrow. Without a continuous supply of replacement cells, the blood counts will fall, because blood cells only live for a short time. Most chemo- therapy drugs temporarily interfere with this replacement process. The temporary falls in blood counts that result can cause serious problems.

Neutrophils

One of the white blood cells normally produced by the bone marrow is the **neutrophil**. Its most important job is to fight off bacteria. Neutrophils last four to five days in the blood normally, and only a few hours if there is a bacterial infection somewhere in the body. The normal total white cell count for an adult is between four and ten thousand cells per cubic millimetre of blood (this is often abbreviated—so if, for example, you are told your white count is four, this means four thousand cells per cubic millimetre). Neutrophils normally make up forty to seventy-five per cent of the total white cells (that is, between two thousand and seven thousand five hundred is a normal neutrophil count).

Chemotherapy doses and programmes are usually designed so that the neutrophil count is unlikely to fall below one thousand per cubic millimetre at any stage. This is because people with counts lower than this can get very serious infections very quickly.

Because there is nothing to stop bacteria from multiplying freely in their blood, life-threatening infections can develop even from bacteria which are harmless for people with normal neutrophil counts. Bacteria that we normally live with quite happily—in the air, on our skins, in our noses, mouths and intestines, can cause death within twenty-four hours if they get into the blood of a person who cannot produce neutrophils. Early signs of such infections include fever, going hot and cold and shivering spells.

The only possible way of controlling infections in people with very few neutrophils is with big doses of intravenous antibiotics to which the bacteria are sensitive. Even then, recovery may not occur unless the bone marrow starts to produce neutrophils quickly.

Platelets

The situation can be equally serious if chemotherapy causes a severe fall in the **platelet** count. The blood cannot clot properly without normal numbers of platelets. The normal platelet count is one hundred and fifty to four hundred thousand per cubic millimetre of blood. Platelets normally last seven to ten days in the blood and for a much shorter time if they are needed to stop bleeding. If the platelet count is less than ten thousand per cubic millimetre of blood, bleeding can occur for no apparent reason. Again, chemotherapy doses and programmes are normally designed so that the platelet count is not likely to fall this low.

Bleeding can take the form of bruising, a rash of spots that don't fade when you press on them, bleeding from the nose, intestines, urinary tract or internal bleeding. Bleeding from the stomach or intestines may appear as vomited blood or brownish material that looks like coffee grounds. Or it may appear in the motions as red blood or as jet black motions. Blood in the urine often looks brown rather than red, something like the colour of black tea. Internal bleeding can cause pain, weakness and dizziness. Bleeding in the brain or its covering can cause headache, vomiting and loss of consciousness. Uncontrolled bleeding from any source can lead to death.

Anaemia

Anaemia (a reduced red blood cell count) is not a frequent or serious side effect of chemotherapy. One reason is because red blood cells live about one hundred and twenty days, very much longer than the five to ten day lifespan of neutrophils and platelets. Most chemotherapy programmes are designed so that the bone marrow is out of action for only a few days at a time, separated by recovery periods. Even in those few days, white cells and platelet counts drop because a large proportion of these short-living cells will die and not be replaced. However, only a small proportion of the long-living red cells die in a few days and they are quickly made up when the marrow recovers. Therefore, any anaemia due to chemotherapy is usually mild and causes only lack of energy, mild weakness and perhaps dizziness. However, chemotherapy can cause substantial drops in the red cell count indirectly as a result of bleeding due to a low platelet count. This can be corrected by transfusion.

Reducing the Chance of Chemotherapy Producing Low Blood Counts

I have told you that, ideally, chemotherapy programmes are planned so that the blood counts are unlikely to fall dangerously low.

If your pre-treatment counts are not normal, your doctor must find out why before starting treatment. Important possibilities include previous radiotherapy or chemotherapy treatment and cancer actually growing in the bone marrow. Radiotherapy permanently damages any marrow that lies with the treated field. In adults, the pelvic bones, spine and upper thighs are the bones which contain most of the blood-producing marrow. Radiation of these areas can therefore cause permanently low blood counts. Most chemotherapy drugs only have a temporary effect on the bone marrow but repeated doses of some can cause permanent damage. These include melphalan, busulphan and the nitrosoureas.

If your marrow has been permanently damaged by previous

treatment or other diseases it would be very dangerous to have the usual doses of chemotherapy. Unfortunately, the doses that are small enough to be safe for you are less likely than the usual doses to damage your cancer cells. Your chances of remission would be much less than for people having full doses, so don't be misled into thinking that overall figures apply in your case. Ask your doctor what *your* chances would be.

A difficult dilemma arises when the cancer itself is the reason for low pre-treatment counts. This happens both with primary cancers of the bone marrow, such as the leukaemias and myeloma and also with secondary cancer in the bone marrow. There is no really safe way of dealing with this situation. Without any treatment the cancer will grow, damaging the marrow even more extensively and causing the blood counts to fall even further. With chemotherapy treatment, the blood counts will also fall, at least to start with. In this case the fall is due to the combined effects of the cancer and the chemotherapy on the bone marrow. Such a fall would not last long *provided* the cancer was sensitive to the treatment. If you have cancer in your marrow and chemo-therapy is recommended, you're between the devil and the deep blue sea. If you don't have any treatment you will die quite soon. If you do, you *could* die (of infection or bleeding) even sooner than you would have without the treatment. Even so, this risk could be worth taking, especially if you have a cancer which is curable, or at least has a good chance of going into remission. You are facing a difficult decision, but you are the best one to make it.

Importance of Blood Tests Before Each Course of Treatment

So far I have been talking mainly about working out doses for the first course of a chemotherapy programme. What actually happens to your blood counts as a result of each course of treatment determines what doses you should have for the next course. Your blood count must be checked, at the very least, immediately before *every* course of treatment. It is extremely dangerous to start a new course of treatment before making quite sure that the marrow has recovered from the previous one. Most chemotherapy drugs produce a typical pattern. However, it is not safe for your doctor to assume that you are following this pattern. Your doctor can't be sure that it is safe for you to start a new treatment course without checking your blood counts. Usually the white cell and platelet counts begin to fall three or four days after treatment, are at their lowest after seven to ten days and back to normal two and a half to three weeks from the beginning of the previous treatment. This is why most treatments are repeated every three to four weeks. A few drugs, for example melphalan and the nitrosoureas also cause a second drop in the white cell and platelet counts four to seven weeks after the last treatment. This is why these drugs are usually repeated only every six to eight weeks.

The absolute minimum that should be checked before each treatment is the total white cell, red cell and platelet counts. Preferably a neutrophil count should also be done. Because they are more sensitive to chemotherapy than some of the other types of white cells, they *can* be very low even when the total white count is normal or near normal. A normal total white count does *not* ensure a normal neutrophil count.

It may be convenient for you to get your blood tested the day before each treatment is due. If you do this, you can be sure that all the results will be ready when you come for your treatment. However, if you prefer to have the blood sample taken and get your treatment at the same visit, you will have to be prepared to wait while your sample is tested. This should only take a few minutes from when the blood reaches the laboratory if you are attending a big clinic or hospital which has a machine for doing all the blood counts. The machine may even be capable of counting each type of white blood cell separately (this is called a differential count). If so, not only your total white cell count but also your neutrophil count should be available within a few minutes of your blood reaching the laboratory. If your counts have to be done by hand they will take longer.

At some clinics which don't have differential white cell counting machines, doctors are prepared to start the next course of treatment without knowing the neutrophil count, as long as the total white cell count is normal or near normal. This is usually safe but not foolproof. If you are attending such a clinic and don't want to run the risk of starting a treatment when your neutrophil count is down you should either have your blood sample taken the day before or be prepared to wait until the neutrophil count is done by hand. Discuss this with your doctor.

Correcting Dangerously Low Blood Counts

Well, we've talked about how to reduce the chance of producing dangerously low blood counts with chemotherapy. What can be done if they do occur anyway?

Transfusion may seem the obvious answer. It certainly is a very good way of dealing with a low red cell count (anaemia). A transfusion will correct this immediately and the transfused red cells will last a month or so. However, there are virtually no platelets or white blood cells in a stored unit of donated blood and very few even in a unit (one pint or six hundred millilitres) of fresh blood. Useful numbers of platelets can be obtained only by separating them from six to eight units of fresh blood (donated the same day). To obtain useful numbers of white blood cells we need fifty to sixty units of fresh blood. This is obviously pretty impractical, especially when you consider that transfused platelets and white cells only last one or two days!

Some clinics and hospitals have a machine called a cell separator which does make platelet and white cell transfusions much simpler for everyone except the donor, who has to remain linked to the machine for some hours. The donor's blood goes out of one vein into the machine, the platelets and/or white cells are separated off and the rest of the blood is returned through another vein. Only a small amount of the donor's blood is in the machine at any one time but over a few hours very large numbers of platelets and white blood cells can be extracted and transfused into the person who needs them. The healthy donor is in no danger because new white cells and platelets from their marrow will quickly replace those that have been removed.

Unfortunately, this cumbersome way of correcting low white cell and platelet counts is a very short-term solution because the transfused white cells and platelets last only a day or two at the most. Unless the donor is identical, the recipient may quickly build up antibodies which destroy the transfused cells within a matter of hours. Such reactions are not usually a problem with red cell transfusions, because there are reliable ways of matching them up and choosing donors whose red cells will not be destroyed by the recipient. It is much more difficult to match white cells and platelets.

Because of the antibody problem, platelet and white cell transfusions are usually recommended only when the patient is bleeding or has a serious infection. While there are no other ways of stopping bleeding due to too few platelets, there are other ways of treating infections due to too few neutrophils. Big doses of intravenous antibiotics to which the bacteria are sensitive are capable of controlling many of these infections without the help of a lot of neutrophils. The earlier treatment starts, the greater its chance of success. If you have fever, hot and cold or shivering spells during chemotherapy, you must notify your doctor immediately.

What about preventing infections? I described protective nursing and its limited benefits on page 224. This is mainly recommended for people with acute leukaemia, who are expected to have low white cell counts continuously over several weeks or months. People with other types of cancer rarely have low white cell counts for more than a few days at a stretch. However, they are often advised to avoid crowded places, and people with sore throats and colds and even the company of small children through-out their chemotherapy. I don't think this is good advice. The fact is that, short of the sterile environment described on page 224, there is no way of avoiding exposure to bacteria which could be harmful to a person with few neutrophils. They are in the air, on your skin, in your nose, mouth and intestines. Why restrict your enjoyment of life when the restrictions will make very little difference to your chance of getting a serious infection? The important precautions are these: *your doctor* can minimise your chances of ever getting a dangerously low count in the first place by planning your treatment carefully. *You* can reduce the chance of any infection developing to a serious stage by reporting to your doctor for tests and treatment as soon as you notice any symptoms of infection.

Nausea And Vomiting

Nausea is feeling squeamish, queasy or sick in the stomach. We all know what vomiting is! Almost every chemotherapy drug can cause nausea and vomiting, but some are much less likely to do so than others. Ones that rarely cause a great deal of nausea include melphalan, chlorambucil, bulsulphan, vincristine, vinblastine, bleomycin, methotrexate and fluorouracil.

Anti-Nausea Medication

Whatever chemotherapy drugs you are having, you need to be prepared for the possibility of nausea. Here's what I suggest if your treatment is on an outpatient basis. For your first course make sure you have some anti-nausea medication on hand, but take them only if you start to feel nauseated. You may not need them. If you do start to feel nauseated take them immediately, rather than wait until you are actually vomiting. It is much easier to control this symptom if you start on it while it is mild.

Your doctor should tell you how frequently you can repeat the anti-nausea medication. Keep taking them at these intervals as long as you feel at all nauseated, unless you are experiencing unpleasant side effects such as drowsiness or restlessness.

If you are dissatisfied with your anti-nausea medication, either because it doesn't work well enough and/or because of side effects, ask your doctor to prescribe a different one for your next course. Different people react differently and it may take a bit of trial and error to find the one that suits you best.

If you are actually vomiting and can't keep an anti-nausea pill down, there are other ways of tackling the problem short of going into hospital. One alternative is to try an anti-nausea medication in suppository form. Several different ones are available. You can insert these into the rectum (back passage) yourself. The medication is absorbed into the bloodstream from there and will do the same job as a pill, sometimes a better one because suppositories usually are longer acting. Another alternative is to arrange for anti-nausea injections at home, given either by a visiting district nurse (if available), friend or even yourself. You can ask to be taught how to give yourself injections if this is the alternative you prefer. It has one big advantage—you can be sure that the person who can give the injection will be there when you need them!

If you are a person who is not particularly distressed by nausea, you may prefer not to take any medication. That's up to you. Some people find that they can settle their stomachs by eating dry foods such as toast or dry biscuits, or with cold drinks such as lemonade. Eat small meals or snacks often and slowly and avoid fatty foods. Lying down after eating (if possible) can also be helpful.

If you feel very anxious about the possibility of nausea, you might prefer to take preventive anti-nausea treatment with your first course of chemotherapy. If you do this—start taking anti-nausea treatment as soon as you have the chemotherapy rather than waiting to see whether nausea develops—then you may be taking the anti-nausea treatment unnecessarily. That doesn't matter as long as it has no side effects. It's up to you whether you take it as prevention or wait until you actually get nausea (if ever).

If your first treatment does cause troublesome nausea, I would definitely suggest taking preventive anti-nausea medication with later courses. Start taking them well before the stage at which you previously experienced nausea.

If you have distressing nausea and vomiting that is not controlled by a variety of anti-nausea medications, another possible solution is to change your chemotherapy treatment. Ask your doctor whether another drug or drugs can be substituted for the one(s) that are producing the nausea. Alternatively, the dose could be reduced or the responsible drug(s) dropped altogether. Ask your doctor how much difference this is likely to make to the outcome of your treatment. You can then decide what is the best course of action for you. You should tolerate serious nausea and vomiting only if your treatment offers a great enough counterbalancing benefit and you are satisfied that there is no better alternative.

Anticipatory Nausea

It is not unusual for people who have had unpleasant nausea with

241

chemotherapy to develop **anticipatory** nausea and vomiting. This means starting to feel ill or even vomiting *before* you get your chemotherapy. If this happens to you, it does *not* mean that you are going crazy or that you are a weak person. It simply means that your body is anticipating your previous unpleasant experiences. You have developed what we call a conditioned response. A nausea response is being triggered not simply by the chemotherapy itself, but also by other things that happen around the same time. Thus, for example, nausea may be triggered off by the sight, smell or even the very thought of your injection or tablets, the clinic, the clinic staff, the clinic car park, or the vehicle in which you usually travel to and from your treatment.

If you are very anxious about your treatment, and/or have developed anticipatory nausea, you could consider learning relaxation techniques and/or taking a mild tranquilliser before your treatment. Both of these approaches can be very helpful. Try not to feel embarrassed about wanting to try them. Your anxiety and/or anticipatory nausea are normal reactions to a very stressful situation. Your doctor should give these problems the same attention as any other aspect of your cancer and its treatment.

Damage To Mucous Membranes

Mucous membranes is a general name for the linings of the mouth, gullet, stomach, intestines and other internal organs. These linings are sensitive to chemotherapy because they contain a high proportion of dividing cells.

For example, the lining of the mouth is normally completely renewed about every twenty-four hours. Many chemotherapy drugs interfere with this process so that, when the old surface cells come off, they are replaced much more slowly than normal. This can cause soreness, unusual sensitivity to hot and cold, and mouth ulcers. The resulting raw, open areas can easily become infected. Fortunately, the whole process usually lasts only a few days to a week during each treatment cycle. This reaction is common with some drugs—for example, methotrexate, fluorouracil, actinomycin D and bleomycin, and rare with others—for example, melphalan, vincristine and cis-platinum. It is a possibility however, with nearly all drugs. The severity and the length of time it lasts depends on the dose.

Mouth reactions usually start within a few days of treatment. You can minimise the problem by taking steps to protect the lining of your mouth from infection or any other irritation. If you are having drugs that are likely to cause mouth ulcers (or actually have caused them on previous treatments) ask your doctor for supplies of antiseptic mouth wash and anti-thrush medication beforehand. Use each of these about four times a day from when your mouth first starts to feel sore until it feels quite normal again. Avoid very hot foods or drinks and keep any dentures out of your mouth as much as possible.

The anti-thrush medication is important because thrush is the most common type of infection in this situation. You may have seen it in babies' mouths. It forms white patches which look a bit like dabs of paint. If a patch is gently scraped off, a raw surface is left. A commonly affected site is under a dental plate. The anti-thrush medications come in syrup or lozenge form. If you are using the syrup make sure you swish it thoroughly around your mouth and keep it there for at least two minutes before swallowing it. It is important to swallow these medications because the thrush can spread down into the throat. Symptoms of this can include soreness and difficulty swallowing.

The treatment I have described is fine for prevention, but often not enough for treatment of an established thrush infection. In this case, it is best to suck anti-thrush lozenges almost continuously, if you can. If this is too painful, use the syrup at least every two hours while you are awake. Soluble aspirin, dissolved in lukewarm water, swished around the mouth and swallowed every few hours is, in my opinion, the most effective way of controlling mouth pain (but you can't do this if your treatment includes methotrexate—see page 264).

If the problems with your mouth or throat are so severe that you are not prepared to go through them again, make this very clear to your doctor. The reaction can be reduced by cutting down the dose of the drug or drugs responsible or even stopping them altogether. Of course, this could mean that your cancer is less likely to be controlled. Weigh the cost against the benefit. You would probably be more likely to put up with severe side effects if this meant a high chance of cure than if you had only a small chance of a short remission.

The lining of the intestines is also quite sensitive to chemotherapy drugs. Symptoms can include a vague stomach ache, crampy pains, wind, and diarrhoea (which can contain blood in very severe cases). Avoid foods which cause wind and cramps, like very spicy foods, beans, cabbage, etc. Eat your food warm rather than hot and try small meals more often. Drink plenty of fluids. If the reaction is so severe that you don't want to go through it again, consider reducing the dose of the responsible drug(s) or even stopping them altogether.

It is unusual to develop symptoms from irritation of other mucous membranes, because they renew their linings less often than the mouth, throat and intestines. Other sites which can be affected, however, include the nose and the vagina.

Interference With Ovarian And Testicular Function

Women

The specialised cells of the ovary are sensitive to many chemotherapy drugs. These drugs can damage both the hormone-producing cells and the ova (eggs). Drugs that are especially likely to interfere with the function of the ovaries include bulsulphan, chlorambucil, cyclophosphamide, melphalan and mustine. However, there is no drug that can be guaranteed not to. There is also no reliable way of preventing these side effects.

If you have already had your menopause, you may not notice any symptoms of ovarian damage. However, if you are still menstruating, your periods may become erratic or stop altogether. You may also experience some of the symptoms which can occur during a normal menopause, such as hot flushes, relative dryness of the vagina, mood swings and loss of interest in sex. You may become infertile (unable to fall pregnant). However, there is no way of definitely telling whether or not you are fertile. Even if you haven't had a period for months, you could still fall pregnant. It is therefore important to take reliable contraceptive precautions anyway.

Chemotherapy and Pregnancy

Any pregnancy conceived *during* chemotherapy is risky. There is definitely a higher than normal risk of miscarriage and of birth defects. We don't know for certain whether or not a pregnancy started *after* completing chemotherapy is more risky than normal. Quite a few women who have had chemotherapy have later produced perfectly normal babies. However, there haven't been enough of these pregnancies for us to know definitely whether or not they carry a higher risk than normal of miscarriage and/or birth defects.

If you do develop symptoms of menopause during chemotherapy, you may still go back to having normal, regular periods later. Periods can start again months or even years after completing chemotherapy. The younger you are and the shorter the duration of your chemotherapy, the more likely your ovaries are to recover. However, I know of no tests which can tell us definitely which women's ovaries will recover. I'm afraid you just have to wait and see.

Hormone Replacement

If your periods do almost or completely stop, ask your doctor about replacement hormones. Your doctor should prescribe very small doses of female hormone to replace those which would normally be produced by your ovary. It is important to take them in monthly cycles so as to imitate natural cycles as closely as possible. Normally functioning ovaries release hormones which cause a build up in the lining of the womb. An egg is released from the ovary in the middle of the cycle. If this egg isn't fertilised, the hormone levels change, causing shedding of the thickened lining of the womb. This shedding produces bleeding—

your monthly period. Hormone pills produce the same build up in the lining of the womb. Stopping the pills results in it being shed just as with a normal period. The big difference is that no egg is released during these artifically produced cycles, so the bleeding which occurs does *not* mean that you have become fertile again.

I know it seems a nuisance to still have to put up with periods when your ovaries aren't working, but this is necessary to keep the lining of your womb healthy. If you took the pills continuously the lining would build up excessively and you would get irregular break-through bleeding. Of course, if your uterus (womb) has been removed, there is no reason to take the hormones in cycles — you can take them every day.

You might think it would be much simpler not to take hormones at all. I recommend that you do take them up to the age of normal menopause (about fifty). As well as keeping the lining of the vagina and uterus healthy and helping you to maintain a normal interest in sex, they will also help to keep your bones strong and to prevent hardening of your arteries.

For those of you who are being treated for breast cancer, the situation is a bit more complicated. Breast cancer cells are often sensitive to the hormonal balance in the body. Breast cancer cells of some young women are actually stimulated to grow by female hormone. The reverse is also true. Remissions of secondary breast cancer can sometimes be produced by removing functioning ovaries — the normal source of female hormone (see pages 292-3 if you want to read more about this). If you have had breast cancer and are less than fifty years old, the benefits of taking female hormone may be outweighed by the fact that they could stimulate any cancer cells that are still in your body.

Men

The testes contain two types of specialised cells — the ones which give rise to sperm and the ones which produce male hormones. The cells which produce sperm are very sensitive to chemotherapy drugs, but the ones which produce male hormones are rarely damaged. This means that most men having chemotherapy maintain a normal interest in sex and can get an erection and ejaculate (come) normally. The ejaculate is of only slightly less than normal volume because most of it comes from the prostate gland, not the testes. However, if examined under the microscope, it would be found to contain very few or no sperm. This means that, although they can have normal sex, men who are having chemotherapy are very unlikely to father children.

After stopping chemotherapy, the testes can recover their ability to produce sperm. This may take some years and is more likely for younger men. There is no way of definitely predicting which men will recover. There is also no reliable way of protecting the testes from damage in the first place.

It is important to realise that, even if your sperm count is known to be extremely low, it is still possible, although unlikely, that you could father a child. This should be avoided *while* you are actually having chemotherapy because pregnancies conceived during this time carry a higher risk of miscarriage and of birth defects than normal. I therefore strongly recommend that you make sure that you or your partner use a reliable contraceptive method while you are having chemotherapy. Once you have completed chemotherapy it is probably not as risky. Certainly some men have fathered perfectly normal children after completing chemotherapy. However, there have not been enough cases for us to know definitely whether or not the risk of miscarriage and birth defects remains a bit higher than normal.

If you are keen to improve your chances of fathering children after chemotherapy, you could consider banking some semen beforehand. Artificial insemination using your semen does not have a good chance of success unless you can store at least six specimens of good quality taken two to three days apart. Therefore, before deciding whether or not to bank some of your semen you should have it tested. The so-called quality is determined by your sperm count and the ability of your sperm to withstand freezing and thawing. Unfortunately, at least at the stage when chemotherapy is being considered, a lot of men with cancer have low counts and/or sperm which don't recover well from freezing. The reasons are not well understood, but poor general health, a high level of stress and recent anaesthetics can all play a part. If your semen is judged to be of poor quality, it is still just possible, but very unlikely, that it could produce a pregnancy when inseminated.

The other factor you should take into account when deciding about storing semen is the importance for you of the resulting two to three week delay in starting chemotherapy. If you have a rapidly growing type of cancer, the number of cells could increase greatly in a few weeks. For example, the chance of curing cancers like choriocarcinoma and Burkitt's lymphoma would be seriously reduced by such a delay.

Increased Risk Of Developing A New Cancer

People who live for some years after treatment of certain types of cancer have an increased risk of developing new cancers. The fact that there is an increased risk is definite but the reasons are not so definite. We do not know how much of it is directly due to the chemotherapy itself. Certainly chemotherapy drugs such as cyclophosphamide, mustine, chlorambucil and melphalan are known to produce a lot of mutations—changes in the genetic make-up of cells which could lead to cancer (I explained a bit about mutations in Chapter 2). Another factor is probably the depression of the immune system that is produced by some chemotherapy drugs and some cancers themselves (especially Hodgkin's disease). When the body's natural defence systems are not working properly, any cancer cell that does develop is more likely to survive and give rise to an actual cancer growth. A third definite factor is radiation treatment. As you know, radiation on its own increases the risk of new cancers. However, the risk is even higher when both radiotherapy and chemotherapy have been used.

Three types of cancer where there is definitely an increased chance of developing a new type of cancer some years after chemotherapy treatment are Hodgkin's disease, multiple myeloma and cancer of the ovary. The risk of acute leukaemia is higher than normal for all three. In the case of Hodgkin's disease, the risk of some other cancers, including non-Hodgkin's lymphoma and skin cancers is also increased.

These three cancers have at least two things in common. They are all cancers that have been successfully treated with chemotherapy for over twenty years. Secondly, many people who have had chemotherapy for these cancers have lived for quite a few years afterwards—long enough to get a new cancer. It is possible that a definitely increased risk of new types of cancer has not been found following treatment of other cancers simply because not enough of these people have lived long enough after their chemotherapy. This could change with the recent increasing use of adjuvant (preventive) chemotherapy (see pages 215–19). A lot of people who are likely to live a long time are now receiving chemotherapy. The possible resulting increased risk of new cancers is particularly worrying when we consider that some of these people do not need the chemotherapy in the first place. I think it is a factor you should take into account when considering adjuvant chemotherapy, especially if the chance of your original cancer recurring *without* adjuvant chemotherapy is not high. Ways of making the risk of second cancers as small as possible are by keeping the duration of treatment short and by avoiding the use of the mutation-producing drugs listed above.

Damage To Tissues At Site Of Injection

Some chemotherapy drugs are very irritating to any tissues with which they make direct contact. These include adriamycin, mustine, actinomycin D, vincristine, vinblastine, mitomycin C, mithramycin and etoposide. The only way you can have these drugs is by an injection directly into the vein. Even when correctly given they can cause soreness and redness along the vein, which may be followed by narrowing or even complete blockage. These reactions are more likely if the vein is a small one. If these drugs leak outside the vein they can cause pain and redness followed by ulceration which will not heal over without the help of a skin graft.

If you are having one of these drugs and the staff are finding it difficult to get needles into your veins, I suggest you seriously consider having a Hickman's catheter (see page 228). With one of these you can be quite sure that the drug is going cleanly into a large vein.

If you don't have a Hickman's catheter, make sure that no one ever injects one of these drugs unless they are watching the point of entry of the needle. If you already have an intravenous drip in your arm, the safest way to have these drugs is by an injection into the tubing, with the point of entry of the needle under constant observation for any signs of leakage. I don't believe it is safe to leave these drugs dripping in unobserved unless the intravenous is very securely placed (like a Hickman's catheter).

Kidney Blockage With Uric Acid

When cells die they release, amongst other things, a substance called uric acid. The body gets rid of the small amounts of uric acid that are normally produced by filtering it out into the urine through the kidneys. If a great number of cancer cells are destroyed in a short time, very large amounts of uric acid are released into the blood. This can result in so much uric acid passing into the urine that it can't all remain dissolved. It then forms a thick sludge which can stop the kidneys from working altogether by blocking up their internal channels. While this situation may be overcome by using dialysis (kidney machines), it often proves fatal.

Because it is a result of the destruction of large numbers of cancer cells within a short time, this side effect can occur only when the cancer cells are very sensitive to the treatment being used. This side effect can be fatal. Death due to kidney blockage with uric acid is a terrible tragedy. I say this for two reasons. Firstly, it is completely preventable. Secondly, the cancers which are so sensitive to chemotherapy that this can happen are often curable ones.

This serious side effect is preventable. Steps should be taken to prevent kidney blockage by uric acid *before* starting treatment on any person who has a lot of rapidly growing cancer cells that are likely to be very sensitive to chemotherapy. Examples include leukaemias and rapidly growing lymphomas such as Burkitt's lymphoma and acute lymphoblastic lymphoma. The main means of preventing kidney blockage are by using a drug called allopurinol and by taking plenty of fluids. Allopurinol helps the body to change uric acid into other substances which dissolve much more easily and therefore will not sludge up the kidneys. Allopurinol comes in tablet form and should, if at all possible, be started at least three days before the chemotherapy. Plenty of fluids should be taken intravenously if nausea or vomiting prevents you from drinking enough. Blood tests should be done at least once a day to check the levels of uric acid and other minerals such as potassium and calcium.

I stress that this problem occurs only when there are large numbers of cancer cells which are extremely sensitive to chemotherapy. This is rarely true for any cancers other than rapidly growing, chemotherapy-curable ones. There is really no need to worry about this complication if you don't have one of these types of cancer.

THE INDIVIDUAL DRUGS

Actinomycin D

You can have this drug only by intravenous injection because it is very irritating to any tissue with which it makes contact (see page 249). It is yellow in colour. Common side effects include nausea, vomiting, hair loss, low blood counts, mouth ulcers and diarrhoea. It can also cause an extensive acne type of rash.

Another side effect is radiation recall. This means that the drug can produce a flare-up of any previous radiation reaction, even when the radiation was given years earlier and the reaction had completely cleared up. Reactions to any radiation that is being given at the same time as this drug are more severe than would otherwise be expected. For example, any skin that has been previously irradiated can become red and sore again. Skin that is irradiated during actinomycin D treatment will show a more severe reaction than otherwise expected. The same thing can happen with internal radiation reactions. For example, a previous reaction in the throat or lungs can flare up again, producing symptoms similar to the original reaction.

Because of this, your doctor should give you a smaller than usual dose of actinomycin D if you have previously had troublesome radiation reactions. Also, any radiation given during actinomycin D treatment must be planned and supervised particularly carefully.

Adriamycin

Adriamycin can only be had by intravenous injection, because it is very irritating to any tissue with which it makes contact (see page 249). Adriamycin is red in colour. The colour can be passed out through the kidneys, so don't be alarmed if your urine temporarily goes bright red after each injection!

The body gets rid of adriamycin by changing it into an inactive form in the liver. It is extremely important that blood tests to check your liver function are done before your dose of adriamycin is calculated. If your liver is not functioning normally, you should have a smaller dose than usual. The usual safe dose of adriamycin would be very dangerous for you because it would cause severe and prolonged drops in white cell and platelet counts which could even prove fatal. All other side effects would also be much worse.

Common side effects include radiation recall (see page 251) fever (within a few hours of injection), skin rashes and gradual darkening of the skin (this takes months and gradually fades when adriamycin treatment is stopped).

A serious and permanent side effect of adriamycin is damage to the heart. Adriamycin can cause weakening of the heart muscle and damage to the electrical system of the heart. Symptoms can include fatigue, palpitations, swelling of the ankles and breathlessness which is typically aggravated by lying down and improved by sitting up. Chest pain is not a symptom of this reaction. A chest X-ray could show an enlarged heart. The electrocardio-graph might be abnormal, but not necessarily.

For an average-sized adult, anything up to about 850 milli-grams of adriamycin in total is very unlikely to produce any serious heart damage. It is unsafe ever to exceed this limit because the risk of heart damage then increases drastically. The spacing of the doses doesn't make any difference to the safe total amount. The risk is much higher for people who already have anything wrong with their heart and for people whose heart has previously received any radiation. The use of cyclophosphamide, actino-mycin D or high-dose methotrexate either before or during adriamycin treatment may also increase the risk. People in these categories must be carefully checked for early signs of heart damage right from the first dose of adriamycin, because no dose is completely safe for them.

Your doctor can check for heart damage in the following ways: by asking you about the symptoms mentioned above, by listening to your heart and lungs with a stethoscope, by checking for swollen ankles, and by arranging chest X-rays, electrocardio-graphs and special forms of radio-isotope scans to check the efficiency of the heart. Unfortunately there are no tests which can be relied on to pick up early heart damage before any symptoms develop.

There are medications which can help the heart to work more efficiently if it is damaged, but any damage is permanent. If you do develop signs or symptoms of heart damage, it is essential that you *never* have any more adriamycin. One more dose at any time, even if it is years later, could cause very serious, even fatal, heart damage.

All of this applies only when adriamycin is given intravenously. There is one other special way of having it. This is in dilute form injected directly into the bladder through a catheter (a plastic tube passed into the bladder through the urinary passage). This method can sometimes control very small bladder cancers. When used in this way, very little of the drug is absorbed into the bloodstream, so general side effects are very unlikely to occur.

Asparaginase

The only type of cancer which this drug has any chance of controlling is acute lymphoblastic leukaemia.

You can have asparaginase either by injection into a vein or into a muscle. It differs from most chemotherapy drugs in that it does *not* cause sore mouth, diarrhoea or hair loss, and has only a slight effect on bone marrow cells. However, it does have a lot of other side effects.

The most worrying are severe allergic reactions occurring within ten to fifteen minutes of injection. Symptoms can include flushing, wheezing, vomiting, faintness due to low blood pressure, and loss of consciousness. This reaction can be fatal. A doctor should give the injection and stay with you for at least half an hour. Medications and equipment to deal with such an emergency should be close at hand. If you experience any of the above allergic symptoms it would be extremely dangerous to have asparaginase ever again.

Another form of allergic reaction—itchy raised hives and weals—is less serious and can often be controlled by anti-histamines.

Other side effects occurring the day of treatment include nausea, vomiting, fever and hot and cold spells.

Asparaginase damages the liver, interfering especially with its job of making blood proteins and substances to help the blood clot normally.

Asparaginase can also damage the pancreas. It can cause acute diabetes, for which insulin injections would be necessary. This is not usually permanent. It can also cause inflammation of the pancreas (pancreatitis) resulting in severe stomach and back pain, vomiting, and fever. If you develop inflammation of the pancreas it is very dangerous to ever have any more asparaginase.

Another problem which asparaginase can produce is brain damage. Sometimes this results only in drowsiness, but confusion, loss of consciousness and fits can occur. These symptoms are not permanent.

Bleomycin

You can have bleomycin either by intravenous or intramuscular injection. A common side effect is fever on the day of injection. This can often be prevented or controlled with aspirin or a drug called indomethacin. Bleomycin can also cause skin rashes and/or darkening of the skin especially in the creases of the elbows and knees. Mouth ulcers are a common side effect. However, it rarely causes hair loss and doesn't damage the bone marrow.

A serious and permanent side effect of bleomycin is lung damage. The symptoms can start weeks or months after having bleomycin. Lung damage is unlikely to develop at total doses of less than about 340 milligrams for an average-sized adult. The risk increases sharply if this limit is passed. The risk is greater if you are over fifty years old, very underweight or have anything else already wrong with your lungs, especially radiation damage. If you fall into any of these categories, you could get lung problems after as little as 100 milligrams of bleomycin.

The only way of avoiding serious damage to the lungs is to pick it up in the early stages and then stop the bleomycin. The earliest symptom is often a dry cough so tell your doctor immediately if you develop one. Shortness of breath and chest pain are later symptoms.

The best way of picking up signs of damage to the lungs early, before symptoms develop, is by doing special breathing tests. The most important one involves checking how much of a gas that is breathed down into the lungs gets through into the bloodstream. This is called either testing the diffusion capacity or the transfer factor. It involves a blood test during the breathing tests. If it is low or falling this means that the lungs are less able to perform the normal job of transferring gases that have been breathed down into the lungs into the bloodstream.

There is no reliable way of preventing or treating this reaction once it has developed. Provided the condition is detected early, and no more bleomycin is given, the reaction should settle down by itself and leave you with only slightly damaged lungs. It is very dangerous to have any more bleomycin at all after a lung reaction has started. This could kill you. At the very least, you would be left with severe and permanent weakening of your lungs. This means you would get puffed out easily, possibly even be short of breath while sitting still, and your lungs would be very prone to infections.

Busulphan

This drug comes in tablet form. Its main side effect is low blood counts. In fact, it is the blood counts that are used to regulate the dose correctly. Busulphan is especially likely to interfere with the function of the ovaries and the testes. Another side effect is darkening of the skin.

The most serious side effect—lung damage—is fortunately very rare. Lung damage due to busulphan can develop many years after taking this drug, as well as during treatment. The symptoms are dry cough and breathlessness. Once it develops, there is no treatment that can correct it and it usually results in death within six months of diagnosis. I stress that this is a *very rare* problem.

Chlorambucil

Chlorambucil comes in tablet form. Common side effects are low blood counts and interference with the function of ovaries and testes.

Most chemotherapy drugs attack only bone marrow cells which are dividing. These cells are quickly replaced when the drug is stopped, restoring the bone marrow completely to normal. In contrast, the marrow is often left permanently damaged after chlorambucil treatment. This is because chlorambucil destroys some of the bone marrow cells which are not dividing, as well as the ones which are. Not all of the non-dividing cells can be replaced. The longer chlorambucil treatment is continued, the greater the risk of permanent damage.

When chlorambucil is being taken in high dose courses with breaks in between, it should be stopped altogether if the blood counts do not come back to something close to normal levels between courses. When chlorambucil is being taken in low doses every day, it should be stopped altogether if the blood counts fall much below normal levels and then fail to return to normal with a break in treatment.

Provided these guidelines are followed, the blood counts after treatment is stopped will be only slightly lower than normal and should cause no symptoms. That's fine as long as you don't want to have more treatment later. However, if you ever do want to have any chemotherapy drug which affects the bone marrow (including chlorambucil itself) again, you must have lower than usual doses. The usual dose would be likely to cause dangerously low counts. Of course, the dose that would be safe for you would not have as good a chance of controlling the cancer as the usual dose. You can minimise your chances of having this problem by taking chlorambucil only for as long as is really necessary and by refusing to take it as part of preventive (adjuvant) treatment.

Cyclophosphamide

You can take cyclophosphamide in tablet form or by intravenous injection. Common side effects include low blood counts, hair loss, nausea and vomiting and interference with the function of the ovaries and testes.

A unique and important side effect of cyclophosphamide is irritation of the lining of the bladder. An active form of this drug is passed out of the body via the kidneys and can damage the lining of the bladder on the way through. The damage can take three forms—acute cystitis, scarring of the bladder and bladder cancer.

Firstly, the symptoms of cystitis (inflammation of the bladder) include burning and stinging while passing urine, a painful dragging feeling in the pelvis and the need to pass urine often, urgently and in small amounts. The symptoms can start within hours, days or weeks of having cyclophosphamide. There is always blood in the urine. Sometimes the blood is in such small amounts that it can only be detected by testing the urine. It is quite common for there to be enough blood for you to see, either as bright blood or just as darkening of the urine. Serious bleeding which is difficult to stop can occur but this is unusual.

The risk of cystitis is highest when cyclophosphamide is given in big doses intravenously, but you can also get it while taking it in tablet form. It is very important to take plenty of fluids while having cyclophosphamide. If you have nausea or vomiting which prevents you from drinking much, you should have intravenous fluids, especially within the first twenty-four hours of a big intravenous dose of cyclophosphamide. A high fluid intake ensures that the active form of the cyclophosphamide is diluted when it passes through the bladder. Empty the bladder often, especially last thing at night and first thing in the morning. The idea is to avoid leaving urine sitting around in your bladder for long periods of time.

Having more cyclophosphamide once the bladder is inflamed can cause very severe cystitis. Sometimes surgery is the only way of stopping the heavy bleeding that can then occur. This means it is very important to act immediately if you get any symptoms of cystitis while taking cyclophosphamide. If it is in tablet form, stop taking them. Notify your doctor. You will need tests to check whether the symptoms are due to infection. If so, antibiotics should clear them up and it would be safe to keep taking your cyclophosphamide. If your symptoms are due to cyclophosphamide, you must *never* have any more. Sometimes another drug such as chlorambucil or melphalan can be substituted for it.

The second type of bladder damage caused by cyclophosphamide is scarring. This can happen with or without previous cystitis. The bladder becomes smaller, so urine may have to be passed in small amounts more often than normal. The longer cyclophosphamide treatment goes on, and the bigger the total dose, the higher the risk. Tests have shown that about half of people who have taken cyclophosphamide for many months or some years have a scarred bladder. However, many of them don't notice any troublesome symptoms.

The third type of bladder problem—bladder cancer—is fortunately unusual. It develops years after cyclophosphamide treatment. Symptoms can be similar to some of those of cystitis— blood in the urine, need to pass urine often and in small amounts and pain or a dragging feeling in the pelvic area. This type of bladder cancer can be hard to diagnose because cells from the bladder lining of anyone who has had cyclophosphamide are not normal and can be confused with cancer cells. If you have a biopsy of your bladder for any reason during or after cyclo- phosphamide treatment, make sure your doctors tell the pathologist (the person who will be examining the specimen under the micro- scope). The pathologist may wrongly diagnose early cancer if he or she doesn't know you have had cyclophosphamide.

Cytosine Arabinoside (Cytosar)

You can have cytosar by any type of injection—intravenous, intramuscular, just under the skin or even into the cerebro-spinal fluid (CSF). Common side efects include low blood counts (including anaemia), nausea and vomiting, diarrhoea and mouth ulcers.

The drug is changed into an inactive form within minutes of getting into the bloodstream. This means that a quick intravenous injection has very little effect. The effect is much greater if the same dose is given in such a way that small amounts are added to the blood continuously over a period of some hours. This can be done with an intravenous drip or by injection into the muscle or under the skin (from whence it will gradually be released into the bloodstream).

As I mentioned above, cytosar can safely be injected into the cerebro-spinal fluid in an attempt to prevent or to treat cancer that is growing there (see page 226). In fact it is probably the *safest* drug for injection into the cerebro-spinal fluid. When it is given this way, very little gets into the bloodstream, so general side effects don't occur. Side effects which can occur, but are rare, include back pain, pains shooting into the arms and legs and pins and needles.

Daunorubicin

This drug is very closely related to adriamycin and has all the same side effects (see page 252). There are three important differences between these two drugs. Firstly, daunorubicin can produce remissions only in leukaemia whereas adriamycin acts against a number of other types of cancer. Secondly, for an average-sized adult, the chance of heart damage with daunorubicin increases sharply over a total dose of about 550 milligrams (it is about 850 milligrams for adriamycin). Thirdly, the dose of daunorubicin does not have to be reduced when the liver is functioning poorly.

D.T.I.C.

This drug's chemical name is so long that most people use just the initials—D.T.I.C. You can have it only by intravenous injection. Common side effects include low blood counts, nausea, vomiting and diarrhoea. A less common side effect is a flu-like reaction with fever, hot and cold spells, muscle pains and just feeling off-colour.

The drug is often given in five day courses repeated once a month, although the benefits and side effects are the same if it is all given in one dose, once a month. Ask your doctor about this if five day courses are recommended for you.

Etoposide (V.P. 16–213)

You can have this drug either by intravenous injection or by swallowing it in capsule or liquid form. When taken by mouth, it is best to take it on an empty stomach. It has a very bitter taste. This can be reduced by mixing it with orange juice or lemonade, neither of which interferes with the action of the drug.

It takes about half an hour to give etoposide intravenously, partly because it takes a large amount of fluid to dissolve it properly and partly because it can cause a drop in blood pressure if it is given too quickly. To get the same effect from a dose taken by mouth, you need about double the intravenous dose. This is because only about half of it is absorbed into the blood from the stomach.

It occasionally produces fever, hot and cold spells, flushing and wheezing. These symptoms are rarely severe but the drug should be stopped if they develop. Antihistamines usually help to clear up these symptoms.

Another uncommon side effect is tingling, numbness or pins and needles in the fingers and toes. This develops only after a number of doses and will disappear provided no more etoposide is given. If you keep having etoposide once these symptoms have started, they will get worse and could be permanent.

Fluorouracil

You can have fluorouracil by intravenous injection or by swallowing it in liquid form. The problem with taking it by mouth is that you can't be sure how much is absorbed into the blood, because it is absorbed erratically. Common side effects include low blood counts, hair loss, nausea and vomiting, mouth ulcers, sore throat and diarrhoea.

It is often recommended that fluorouracil or its close relative, fluoro-deoxyuridine (F.U.D.R.) are given by injection into an artery. The theoretical reason for this is that these drugs are quickly changed into inactive forms by the liver. Injecting them directly into an artery that leads to the target cancer means they go through the cancer before getting to the liver. Unfortunately this advantage is purely a theoretical one while the disadvantages are real. The cancers for which this has been tried are ones where chemotherapy makes no difference to the average length of life—cancers of the colon, pancreas, tongue, and throat. Giving ineffective drugs through an artery doesn't magically make them effective. They still produce only occasional, short remissions and they still make no difference to the average length of life. Against this lack of real advantages you should weigh these real disadvantages—treatment into the artery is more dangerous (because of the risk of heavy bleeding) and much more difficult. If the artery is internal, as it is in the case of colon and pancreas cancers, an operation can even be necessary to put the needle in place!

Hexamethylmelamine

There is no type of cancer that has a good chance of being controlled by hexamethylmelamine. The drug comes in tablet form. Common side effects are nausea, vomiting, loss of appetite, diarrhoea and cramping stomach pains. Low blood counts are also common. If the drug is taken every day for some months, it can cause nerve and brain damage. The symptoms can include pins and needles or numbness in the fingers and toes, sleepiness, depression and loss of balance. These symptoms usually disappear if the drug is stopped.

Hydroxyurea

The only type of cancer which has a good chance of being controlled by hydroxyurea is chronic myeloid leukaemia. This drug comes only in tablet form. Its only common side effect is low blood counts, which go back to normal very quickly when the drug is stopped. Uncommon side effects include nausea, vomiting, sore mouth, diarrhoea, skin rashes and loss of hair.

Melphalan

This is usually taken by mouth but an intravenous form is available. It often damages the ovaries and testes. Hair loss, mouth ulcers, nausea and diarrhoea are all uncommon side effects of melphalan.

The most common and troublesome side effect is low blood counts. Melphalan causes two falls in blood counts, one after a week or two, and another four to six weeks after treatment. It is not safe to take the next course until your counts have recovered from the second fall. This means that if you are having it in short, high dose courses, there must be at least a six week break between courses. Although a blood count taken after four weeks may well be normal, it would still be dangerous to take another course then. If you did, the early drop in blood counts due to the new course would probably happen at the same time as the delayed one from the previous course. This would result in dangerously low counts.

Melphalan damages some bone marrow cells which are not dividing, as well as ones which are. In this respect it is like chlorambucil. If you are considering having melphalan treatment, read the section about the results of damage to non-dividing marrow cells on p 256.

Methotrexate

You can have methotrexate as tablets or by intravenous or intramuscular injection. There are also two special ways of having it that I will describe later in this section. These are high-dose methotrexate and injections of methotrexate into the cerebro-spinal fluid.

Injections are necessary only for doses of methotrexate that are greater than about 50 milligrams for an average sized adult. Smaller doses are reliably absorbed into the system from the stomach. Even if your dose is higher, you can still take it by mouth if you wish, as long as you split it into doses that are each less than 50 milligrams and take them about two hours apart.

Common side effects of usual dose methotrexate include low blood counts and sore mouth. Less common are loss of hair, nausea, diarrhoea, skin rashes and liver damage. Liver damage, which leaves the liver permanently scarred, is more likely if methotrexate is taken every day, rather than in short courses with breaks in between. It is also more common in people who drink a lot of alcohol. There are no blood tests which can be relied on to pick up the permanent type of liver damage. You can reduce your chances of getting it by keeping your alcohol intake down and refusing to take it in small doses every day.

The body has no way of changing methotrexate into an inactive form. The only way it can get rid of it is by passing it out in the urine via the kidneys. This means it is essential that your kidney function is checked before every course of methotrexate treatment. A dose that is quite safe for a person with normal kidneys could kill you if your kidneys were not working normally. This is because the damage done by methotrexate depends on how long it is active in the body.

There are a number of medications which can stop even

perfectly normal kidneys from getting rid of methotrexate quickly. These include aspirin, indomethacin, diphenylhydantoin, and certain antibiotics—sulpha drugs, tetracyclines and chloramphenicol. It is dangerous to take any of these drugs while you are having methotrexate. At the very least, you will get much worse mouth ulcers and much lower blood counts than you would otherwise. Not all doctors know about this. *You* make sure that, while taking methotrexate, you don't take any of the above antibiotics or any painkiller that contains aspirin. Aspirin is in a lot of painkillers. Another name for it is salicylate (s). Check the label for the contents of any painkiller or tablet for arthritis that you take. Ask your doctor whether it contains aspirin if you are not sure. Paracetomol is a safe alternative.

Although the body cannot inactivate methotrexate itself, there is a chemical that can. Folinic acid (also called citrovorum factor or leukovorin) is an antidote to methotrexate. It comes both in tablet and injection form. It should not be needed when methotrexate is taken in the usual dose by people whose kidneys are functioning normally.

High-dose Methotrexate

It *is* needed when methotrexate is used in extremely high doses. In fact, it was the availability of this antidote that led to the development of **'high-dose' methotrexate** treatment. High-dose methotrexate treatment is expensive, complicated and dangerous. You would need to be very sure that there were counterbalancing benefits for you before agreeing to have it. Osteogenic sarcoma (a type of bone cancer) is the only type of cancer where high-dose methotrexate definitely has a greater anti-cancer effect than the much safer usual doses of methotrexate. However, even high-dose methotrexate cannot produce cures in this type of cancer once it has formed definite secondary growths.

There are other types of cancer such as melanoma, mouth and throat cancer and lung cancer where high-dose methotrexate *may* produce temporary remissions slightly more often than usual dose methotrexate. However, it makes no difference to the average length of life. These cancers are simple not very sensitive to *any* chemotherapy drugs, and this includes high-dose methotrexate.

High dose methotrexate would more accurately be called massive dose methotrexate— the doses used can be five hundred or more times the usual safe dose of methotrexate! *Each dose* would well and truly kill you if *all* the precautions listed below are not carefully and exactly observed.

First of all, neutralising doses of folinic acid must be taken every six hours until the amount of methotrexate in the blood drops below a certain level. If nausea or vomiting prevents you from taking the pills, you must have it by injection. You will need the folinic acid for at least three days and possibly much longer. The first few times you have high-dose methotrexate, the amount of methotrexate in the blood should be checked frequently. The doctors will then know how quickly you get rid of it and can work out for how long you must take the folinic acid. It is safe to assume that you will take about the same time to get rid of the same dose of methotrexate in later treatments, *provided* you observe *all* the other precautions listed below for *every* treatment.

Secondly, you must be sure to pass at least three litres of urine per day until you have got rid of the methotrexate. If nausea or vomiting prevents you from drinking plenty of fluids, you must have them intravenously. This is *absolutely essential*. The huge amounts of methotrexate that will be passing through your kidneys need plenty of fluid to keep them dissolved.

It is also essential to keep the urine alkaline (the opposite of acid) until you have got rid of the methotrexate. Methotrexate dissolves much more easily in alkaline than in acid urine. The urine can be made alkaline by taking sodium bicarbonate. You can have this intravenously or in capsule form. You can also help to keep the urine alkaline by avoiding acidic drinks such as orange juice. You (or the staff if you are in hospital) should check the acidity of your urine frequently and take as much sodium bicarbonate as is necessary to keep it alkaline. If you are not staying in hospital, you must learn to test your urine yourself. This involves dipping a specially treated strip of plastic into your urine and then checking its colour against a chart printed on the side of the bottle that the strips come in. The colour of the strip tells how acid or alkaline the urine is. The nursing staff will tell you what colour to aim for.

If you don't pass enough urine and/or if your urine is acid, the methotrexate will not stay dissolved in the kidneys. It will form a sludge which will completely block them. This is extremely serious because, of course, once your kidneys are blocked your body can only get rid of the rest of the methotrexate extremely slowly. Large amounts of folinic acid would be needed for a long time and even then you could die as a result of this complication.

Lastly, it is especially important to avoid the drugs I listed earlier which interfere with the elimination of methotrexate. Even one dose of aspirin can make a big difference.

I'll just repeat here that all these precautions and my warnings about danger apply only to *high-dose* methotrexate. Provided your kidneys are working normally, usual doses of methotrexate (up to 90 or 100 milligrams per dose) are very safe and have few side effects.

Methotrexate Injections Into the Cerebro-Spinal Fluid

The other special way of having methotrexate is by injecting it directly into the cerebro-spinal fluid (see page 226). This may be recommended for prevention or treatment of cancer in the meninges. When given this way, some methotrexate gets out of the cerebro-spinal fluid into the blood, so it can still cause nausea, vomiting, low blood counts and mouth ulcers. Other side effects of injections by lumbar puncture include headache, back pain, stiffness, shooting pain, pins and needles, or weakness in one or both legs.

Whichever way it is given, repeated methotrexate in the cerebro-spinal fluid can also cause headaches, sensitivity to light, fever, drowsiness, loss of balance, fits and even complete loss of consciousness and death. This can happen whether the methotrexate is given by lumbar puncture, through an Ommaya-type reservoir or even as high dose methotrexate. When methotrexate is given in usual doses none gets into the cerebro-spinal fluid. However the amount of methotrexate in the blood with high-dose methotrexate is so great that it does penetrate into the brain and cerebro-spinal fluid. Permanent and even fatal brain damage has occurred in some people who have had repeated high-dose methotrexate and/or injections of methotrexate into the cerebro-spinal fluid. The risk is higher in people who have had radiation treatment to the brain as well.

Mithramycin

You can have mithramycin only by intravenous injection. It causes serious problems if it leaks outside the vein (see page 249). When mithramycin is used as an anti-cancer drug, common side effects include loss of hair, low blood counts, nausea and vomiting, sore mouth, diarrhoea, liver damage and kidney damage and bleeding. Bleeding or easy bruising can be due either to a low platelet count and/or to liver damage. The liver normally produces many of the chemical substances that are necessary for blood to clot normally. Mithramycin can stop the liver from producing these substances.

The only type of cancer which has any chance of being controlled by mithramycin is cancer of the testis. As there are many drugs which are more likely than mithramycin to control this type of cancer, I would never recommend its use as an anti-cancer drug myself.

It does have another use, however, for which I would recommend it. Mithramycin can be relied on to reduce high blood calcium levels in any type of cancer. The doses that will do this are much smaller than the doses needed for an anti-cancer effect. Side effects other than those due to it leaking outside the vein are uncommon and mild with these small doses. The calcium level should stay down for seven to ten days after a dose of mithramycin. See page 134 for more information about the symptoms of, and treatment for, too much calcium in the blood.

Mitomycin C

There is no type of cancer that has a good chance of being controlled by mitomycin C. This drug comes only as an intravenous injection. It damages the tissues if it leaks outside the vein (see page 249).

A common and important side effect is bone marrow damage. Mitomycin C can cause drops in white cell and platelet counts at any time within eight weeks of a dose. This means that there should be six to eight weeks between doses. Permanent bone marrow damage is also common because mitomycin C can destroy even non-dividing bone marrow cells. These cells may not be replaced when mitomycin C treatment stops, leaving the marrow permanently unable to keep white cell and platelet counts at normal levels.

Other side effects include nausea, vomiting and fever. Less common side effects include lung, kidney and liver damage.

We can get rid of some mitomycin C by changing it into inactive forms in the liver. The rest is passed out in the urine. If your liver and/or kidney are not functioning normally, it would not be safe to have the usual dose of mitomycin C.

Mustine

Mustine comes only in injection form. It severely damages the tissues if it leaks outside the vein (see page 249).

Common side effects include hair loss, low blood counts, nausea and vomiting, sore mouth, diarrhoea and interference with the function of the testes and ovaries.

Nitrosoureas

This name covers a group of drugs, each of which have such long chemical names that they are usually referred to just by the initials of those names, such as B.C.N.U. and C.C.N.U.

These drugs commonly cause nausea and vomiting and low blood counts. They can damage non-dividing bone marrow cells. They produce two falls in the white cell and platelet counts— the first one or two weeks after treatment and the second four to six weeks after treatment. Their effects on bone marrow are similar to those of melphalan and chlorambucil. Read page 256 if you are considering having one of these drugs.

Unlike most chemotherapy drugs, these three drugs are all able to penetrate into the brain when used in normal dosage.

(Cis) Platinum (D.D.P)

This drug is often referred to simply as platinum but it is actually a chemical compound of the metal platinum. It is also sometimes referred to by the initials of its full chemical name—D.D.P.

You can have it only by intravenous injection. Common side effects are nausea and vomiting, low blood counts (including anaemia), kidney damage and partial deafness.

There are two reasons why it is essential to check that the kidneys are working normally before *every* dose of cis-platinum. Firstly, the body probably has no way of changing cis-platinum into an inactive form. It can get rid of it only through the kidneys. Secondly, cis-platinum itself can damage the kidneys. If they are not working very efficiently in the first place, a vicious circle results. The cis-platinum is not eliminated quickly and so causes more severe side effects, including more severe kidney damage, which means it is eliminated even less efficiently!

This can be avoided by making sure that the kidneys are functioning normally before every treatment. You will probably get severe and permanent kidney damage if you have cis-platinum when your kidneys are not functioning normally. It is also important to make sure that you can pass at least three litres of urine within the first twenty-four hours of starting your cis-platinum. You should take plenty of fluids and also a drug to help you pass large amounts of urine *before*, during and after having the cis-platinum. It will then be washed quickly through your kidneys.

Cis-platinum is normally given by an intravenous drip over six to eight hours. It is likely that you will have to get most of your fluids this way as well, because nausea and vomiting are so common with cis-platinum. It is dangerous to remove your intravenous drip before you are able to drink normally.

If you do get kidney damage, it will probably be permanent. However, provided the above precautions are taken, any permanent kidney damage should be so mild that you would experience no symptoms from it.

Cis-platinum treatment can also interfere temporarily with the kidneys' ability to correctly regulate the amount of calcium and magnesium in the blood. If there is too little calcium and/or magnesium in the blood, you may have painful spasms of the hands and feet and even fits. These complications should be prevented by checking the amount of calcium and magnesium in your blood regularly. If there is too little, it can be corrected by having extra calcium or magnesium in tablet or injection form.

Cis-platinum can also affect your hearing and/or cause ringing in the ears. You should have hearing tests before starting treatment to make sure your ears are normal to start with, and to get results with which later tests can be compared. Provided you are tested before every second dose, any minor damage should be picked up before you are aware of it. Once there is any sign of damage, further doses will probably make it worse. You will have to weigh this cost against the benefits to decide whether or not to stop your cis-platinum treatment. You might be more prepared to accept partial hearing loss if you have a good chance of complete cure of your cancer than if you have only a small chance of a temporary remission.

There are some antibiotics which should not be used if you are having cis-platinum because they increase the chance of both kidney and ear damage. The most important one is called gentamycin.

Allergic reactions are an uncommon but dangerous side effect of cis-platinum. If they are going to occur, they usually do so within minutes of starting it. Symptoms can include wheezing, swelling of the face, palpitations, faintness, dizziness and loss of consciousness. Your treatment should not be started without a doctor and emergency equipment and drugs close by.

Cis-platinum is sometimes recommended in five day courses. The same total can safely be taken in one dose. This works just as well and has the big advantage of causing nausea and vomiting on only one day instead of five! Ask your doctor about this if five day courses are recommended for you.

Prednisone

Prednisone is actually a hormone but, because it is often used with chemotherapy drugs, most of you would naturally look for it in this chapter. I have described its uses and side effects on pages 286–90 of Chapter 11, so check there if it has been recommended for you.

Procarbazine

This comes in tablet form. Common side effects include nausea, vomiting and loss of appetite. These often improve within a few days, in spite of continuing the procarbazine. It also causes low blood counts.

It is one of the few chemotherapy drugs which penetrates easily into the brain. This may partly account for its side effects of drowsiness, confusion, difficulty with balancing, feelings of restlessness, irritability or over-excitement.

Procarbazine increases the effects of some sedatives and of alcohol. If you wish to take these while having procarbazine, try them in smaller amounts than usual until you see how you react to them. You could experience symptoms like flushing, sweating, and dizziness after quite small amounts of alcohol. It will be several weeks after stopping the procarbazine before this effect disappears.

Streptozotocin

Streptozotocin is actually a nitrosourea, but I have listed it separately because it is quite different to the ones I described on page 268. The only types of cancer that it is likely to temporarily control are very rare cancers of the pancreas (islet cell tumours). You can have it only by intravenous injection.

Nausea and vomiting are common. It has very little effect on the blood counts. Its most serious side effect is kidney damage. It damages only a particular specialised part of the kidneys, resulting in excessive loss of certain proteins and minerals. Only very tiny amounts of these proteins and minerals normally get into the urine. Special blood and urine tests must be done regularly to check for early signs of kidney damage. If streptozotocin is continued once kidney damage has started, it will cause severe and permanent kidney damage which could even kill you. You can reduce the risk of kidney damage by taking plenty of fluids to make sure that you pass plenty of urine and so wash the streptozotocin quickly through the kidneys. You should not have it at all if your kidneys are not normal to start with.

Streptozotocin can also temporarily cause diabetes, for which you could need insulin.

Teniposide (VM-26)

This drug does not have a good chance of controlling any type of cancer. You can have it only by intravenous injection. Teniposide damages the tissues if it leaks outside the vein (see page 249). Common side effects include loss of hair, nausea and vomiting, and low blood counts.

Thioguanine

Leukaemias, especially acute myeloblastic leukaemia, are the only types of cancer likely to be controlled by thioguanine. You can have it as tablets or by intravenous injection.

Common side effects include nausea, sore mouth, diarrhoea and low blood counts, including anaemia.

The body gets rid of thioguanine by changing it into an inactive form in the liver. If your liver is not working normally, usual doses of thioguanine could cause dangerously low blood counts. You would need to have smaller than usual doses.

Thiotepa

This comes as an intravenous injection. Its main side effect is low blood counts. It also interferes with the function of the ovaries and testes. It rarely causes nausea.

The body can get rid of it only through the urine, because it has no way of changing it into an inactive form. This means that it is safe to have it in the usual dose *only* if your kidneys are working normally.

Vinblastine

Vinblastine comes as an intravenous injection. It irritates the tissues if it leaks outside the vein (see page 249). Vinblastine is changed into an inactive form by the liver. It is very important to make sure your liver is functioning normally before having vinblastine. The usual doses of vinblastine cause much more severe side effects in a person whose liver does not function normally. Vinblastine's main side effects are low blood counts and damage to nerves. Another common reaction is aches and pains in the muscles of the back, arms and legs a few days after having vinblastine. These pains can be very extensive and severe, but rarely last more than a few days.

The nerves which are most often damaged are the ones that control the function of the bowel and bladder. Five to ten days after having vinblastine you could get aching or cramping pains all over the stomach area, nausea, vomiting and severe constipation. The risk of having this reaction can be reduced by making sure that the bowel is emptied before having each dose of vinblastine and then taking a low fibre diet and regular laxatives (medications to move the bowels). You should also make sure you take plenty of fluids. If you do get very constipated, you will probably need a number of enemas as well as regular laxatives to get the bowels working again.

If the nerves to the bladder are damaged, you would not be sure when you needed to empty your bladder, it would be hard to get started and hard to empty the bladder completely. You might even be unable to pass urine at all. In this case, a catheter (soft plastic tube) would have to be inserted through the urinary passage into the bladder to drain it, until it started working properly again. Other possible results of nerve damage from vinblastine include pins and needles and tingling in the fingers and toes, unstable blood pressure and impotence.

All of these reactions are temporary, *provided* no more vinblastine is given until things are back to normal. If, for example, you have another dose of vinblastine when you are still very constipated, you could be left with a permanently sluggish bowel. The higher the dose, the closer together the doses and the older you are, the more common and severe are problems due to nerve damage. Nerves which have already been weakened or damaged by something else are especially sensitive to vinblastine. For example, if vinblastine is used soon after an operation during which some nerves were bruised or cut, the consequences could be permanent.

Vincristine

Vincristine is closely related to vinblastine. It also causes serious problems if it leaks outside the vein (see page 249) and it is also changed into an inactive form by the liver. It differs from vinblastine in that it has very little effect on blood counts.

Its main side effect is nerve damage. It can produce all the symptoms of vinblastine nerve damage—see above. The most common forms of nerve damage in the case of vincristine are constipation and pins and needles, tingling or numbness in the fingers and toes. Bladder and other problems are quite uncommon. As long as your only symptoms of nerve damage are mild, temporary constipation and/or mild tingling or numbness in the fingers and toes, further doses of vincristine are unlikely to cause permanent or serious problems. However, if you have any loss of strength at all in the arms or legs, further vincristine will cause more serious and prolonged, even permanent weakness. The movements that are usually affected first are the ability to lift the foot or the wrist. So, for example, if your feet are dragging at all when you walk, or if your grip is weakened, tell your doctor before you have any more vincristine. Find out what difference it is likely to make if you stop having vincristine and balance the likely cost against the likely benefits.

Vindesine

This drug is related to vinblastine and vincristine. It also damages tissue if it leaks outside the vein (see page 249). It produces low blood counts like vinblastine. It also damages the nerves. Read pages 273–74 for information about nerve damage.

Chapter 11

HORMONE TREATMENT

HORMONES AND CANCER TREATMENT

First of all, just what are hormones? Hormones are substances that are produced by certain glands in our bodies for the benefit of other parts of our bodies. They act, not where they are produced, but on other parts of the body, which they reach through the bloodstream. For example, female hormone is produced mainly by the ovaries, but acts on the uterus, breast, skin, bones and other tissues.

Hormones are important in regard to cancer because there are some types of cancer whose growth can be stimulated by certain hormones and inhibited by others. These cancers can sometimes be temporarily controlled by changing the hormone balance so that it is less favourable for them. They include breast cancer, prostate cancer, cancer of the uterus (womb), thyroid cancer, lymphocytic lymphomas and leukaemias, Hodgkin's disease, multiple myeloma and others.

BENEFITS OF HORMONE TREATMENT

Hormone treatments can produce temporary remissions of some cancers but I am afraid that *no* hormone treatment can completely and permanently cure *any* type of cancer. Remissions brought about by changing the hormone balance are always temporary. There are no exceptions to this rule. This is because cancers which start off being sensitive to the hormone balance always finish up losing that sensitivity. Sooner or later, they all develop the ability to grow vigorously, regardless of the hormone balance.

276

Don't let the fact that they cannot cure you put you off seriously considering hormone treatments if you have a hormone-sensitive type of cancer which has spread. Most of these cancers cannot be cured by chemotherapy either. Some of them have a much better chance of going into remission with hormone treatments than with chemotherapy — for example, prostate and uterine cancers. The costs of hormone treatments tend to be less than the costs of most chemotherapy treatments. You may well decide that the cost-benefit balance of a hormone treatment is better than any other available treatments.

You may be advised to have a hormone treatment at the time of surgical removal or radiation treatment of a primary cancer. For example, some doctors recommend removal of the ovaries at the time of treatment of primary breast cancer. Another common recommendation is for female hormone treatment at the time of treatment of primary prostate cancers. Such treatment makes no difference either to the chance of being completely cured or to the average length of life. If there are still some cells in your body after treatment of your primary cancer, hormone treatment will not get rid of them. The only benefit of such treatment is that it may delay recurrence, but it will not prevent it. Hormone treatment at the time of treatment of primary cancer has all the disadvantages of chemotherapy given at this time (see pages 215–18). Only a few people get a small benefit (delay of recurrence) while everyone pays a price.

COST OF HORMONE TREATMENT

Hormones have a beneficial effect only as long as they are present in the right amounts. Either too much or too little of any hormone can have unpleasant and even harmful effects. You will find this explained in more detail later in this chapter under the heading of each individual hormone.

Some hormone treatments interfere with the balance of more than one hormone, not just the one that influences the growth of the cancer. Examples include removal of the adrenal or pituitary glands (see pages 293–95). These treatments carry a higher cost than treatments which alter the amounts of only one hormone. All the ways of changing the hormone balance to treat cancer are described later in this chapter but first of all, let's look at the individual types of cancer concerned.

HORMONE-SENSITIVE CANCERS

Breast Cancer

Breast cancer is often sensitive to the balance of sex hormones in the body. Women who are still having periods tend to have breast cancers which are stimulated to grow by female hormone. Remissions may be produced by reducing the amount of female hormone in the body or by taking male hormone. Women who have had their menopause tend to have breast cancers which can react favourably to a change in the hormone balance in either direction. These women may get remissions by taking female hormone, anti-female hormone, male hormone, corticosteroids (adrenal hormones) aminoglutethimide or having the adrenal glands or pituitary gland removed. Breast cancer in men (yes, men do occasionally get breast cancer) is even more likely than women's breast cancers to be sensitive to the hormone balance. Treatments which may bring about a remission include female hormone, anti-female hormone, corticosteroids, aminoglutethimide and removal of the testes or adrenal glands.

Overall, for women with secondary breast cancer, hormone treatments have about a one in three chance of bringing about a remission whereas for combination chemotherapy treatments the chance of remission is about two in three. However, the overall figures are not very important for you, because there are ways of picking which individuals are likely to react favourably to hormone treatments. Here are the important indicators.

The first is your age—the older you are and the longer the time since your menopause (if you have had it), the more likely that your cancer will be sensitive to the hormone balance.

278

Next is the time between treatment of your primary breast cancer and diagnosis of secondary breast cancer. The longer this is, the more likely that your cancer will be sensitive to the hormone balance. If you already had secondary cancer when your primary cancer was first diagnosed, the chance of it responding to hormone treatment is small.

The location of your secondary cancer is another important indicator. You are most likely to react favourably to hormone treatments if it is in the skin, lymph nodes or pleura (lining of the lung). If it is in the liver or brain it is very unlikely to be sensitive. Bones and lungs are in between.

If you have already reacted favourably to one hormone treatment but your cancer is now active again, treatment has about a one in two chance of bringing about a further remission.

The last important indicator is the presence of what we call oestrogen receptors in your actual cancer. These cannot be checked with a blood test. To find out whether or not your cancer has them, they must test a small sample from the cancer itself (either the primary or a secondary deposit). This is a test that your doctor has to ask for specially, so it is not always done at the time of diagnosis of your primary cancer. If your cancer has plenty of oestrogen receptors there is about a one in two chance that it is sensitive to the hormone balance. If it has hardly any or no oestrogen receptors the chance is less than one in twenty.

Ask your doctor about the alternatives if a hormone treatment is recommended for you. There is always more than one way of changing the hormone balance and you should choose the one that seems best for you. If you do get a remission you may be able to get further remissions when you relapse by having different hormone treatments in turn. Sooner or later your cancer will become unresponsive to the hormone balance but this can take quite a few years.

Cancer Of The Uterus (Womb)

If you have secondary cancer of the uterus, you have about a one in three chance of getting a remission by taking progesterone-type female hormone (see pages 284–85). You are very unlikely to get a remission by changing the hormone balance in any other way.

Prostate Cancer

If you have secondary prostate cancer in your bones, you have about a two in five chance of getting a temporary remission by either having your testes removed or by taking female hormones. There is also about a two in five chance that your cancer will stabilise so that it stops growing for a while but doesn't actually get definitely smaller. Your symptoms will probably temporarily improve if this happens. There is only about a one in five chance that your cancer will show no reaction to one of these hormone treatments.

The chance of getting a remission is about the same whether you have your testes removed or take oestrogen-type female hormone. It is not improved by doing both at the same time. Read pages 282–84. You will see that the side effects of taking oestrogens are far greater than of having your testes removed, but it is up to you to decide which you prefer. Try not to let your natural reluctance to have your testes removed blind you to the disadvantages of oestrogen treatment. Remember that with either treatment you are very likely to be impotent (unable to get an erection) and to lose interest in sex.

Prostate cancer is very unlikely to react favourably to a second hormone treatment. This is true, whether the second treatment is being tried after the first treatment fails to bring about a remission or whether it is tried when you relapse after having had a remission.

Thyroid Cancer

Some types of well-differentiated thyroid cancer (papillary and follicular types) are stimulated to grow by a hormone called thyroid stimulating hormone (T.S.H. for short). This hormone is released by the pituitary gland only when there is not enough thyroid hormone in the blood. Taking extra thyroid hormone is a good way of making sure that your pituitary gland doesn't release any T.S.H. This may reduce your chance of getting a recurrence or at least delay any recurrence.

I can't tell you how much difference the extra thyroid hormone makes, because almost everyone who has been treated for primary thyroid cancer needs to take it anyway. This is because most people treated for primary thyroid cancer are left without any thyroid tissue. It is all either removed surgically or destroyed with radioactive iodine. If this includes you, you must take thyroid hormone anyway. There is no other part of your body that can produce it and it is a hormone that is essential for general good health (see pages 291–92 of this chapter).

Cancers Arising From The Lymphoid/ Plasma Cell Family

The growth of some of these cancers can be inhibited by taking extra corticosteroid hormones (see pages 286–90). They include acute lymphablastic leukaemia, chronic lymphocytic leukaemia, Hodgkin's disease, most non-Hodgkin's lymphomas and multiple myeloma. Corticosteroids on their own will produce only temporary remissions of these cancers. Combining corticosteroids with chemotherapy produces more frequent and longer remissions than when either hormones or chemotherapy are used on their own. The addition of corticosteroids to chemotherapy also has the advantage of reducing some of the side effects of chemotherapy, especially its effect on the bone marrow.

Other Cancers

There are a few other types of cancers which are occasionally sensitive to the balance of sex hormones. These include melanoma and cancer of the kidney (Grawitz tumour). The chance of these cancers going into remission with hormone treatment is very small, well under one in twenty.

We will now look at the various ways of changing the hormone balance. Many different hormones with different names are used in cancer treatment. Often the same hormone is produced by a number of drug companies, each of which give it a different company name (the proprietary name). I will only list the chemical names of some of the most commonly used hormones here. If you can't find the name of the hormone which has been recommended for you, ask your doctor what its chemical name is and what type of hormone it is. If you're still not sure, you could show your doctor this book and ask him or her to indicate which section covers the recommended treatment.

CHANGING THE HORMONE BALANCE BY HAVING TABLETS OR INJECTIONS

Oestrogen-Type Female Hormones

eg: diethyl stilboestrol (stilboestrol),
     ethinyloestradiol and others

All of us, including women who have long passed their menopause and even men, normally have some oestrogens in our bodies. These hormones are produced by the adrenal glands as well as by the ovaries. Taking extra oestrogens in tablet or injection form is a way of producing remissions in men with prostate or breast cancer and in women with breast cancer who are well past the menopause. Oestrogens are likely to stimulate the growth of breast cancer of women who are still having periods, so avoid taking them if you fit this category.

Taking extra oestrogens can cause nausea and vomiting. This side effect is less likely and less severe if you start with a small dose and build it up gradually over several weeks.

Extra oestrogens reduce the body's ability to get rid of salt and water. Because of this they can cause swelling of the ankles, weight gain, and shortness of breath, which is usually worst when lying flat. These symptoms can be corrected by taking fluid tablets to help you get rid of more salt and water. Medications to help the heart work more efficiently may also be needed. Oestrogens can also both cause and aggravate high blood pressure, so your blood pressure should be checked regularly while you are taking them.

Another side effect of extra oestrogens is that they make the blood clot more easily than normal. If you take extra oestrogens you will have a higher chance than normal of getting clots in the veins (thrombosis), and clots travelling through the blood to the lungs. Blood clots in the lungs can cause coughing of blood, sharp chest pain and shortness of breath. When your blood is clotting more readily than normal, strokes and heart attacks are also more likely to happen. All of these complications can be fatal. In fact, the risk of dying from these can be so high that it outweighs any advantage gained by temporarily controlling the cancer.

The risk of serious blood clotting problems depends on the dose of oestrogens. For men, less than the equivalent of three milligrams a day of stilboestrol is probably safe. The safe dose for women is not definitely known but is probably quite a bit higher.

Oestrogens also weaken small blood vessels. You are likely to bruise easily if you take them.

Extra oestrogens cause some special problems for women. You could develop a need to pass urine frequently and/or loss of control of the bladder when coughing, sneezing, laughing etc. If you have not had your uterus removed, you could also experience bleeding from the vagina. This can happen either after you have been taking oestrogens for a long time or when you stop taking them. If the bleeding is heavy, doesn't stop by itself or happens more than once, you can't take it for granted that it is simply due to your oestrogen treatment. You should consider having a curette in order to be sure of the reason for such bleeding. A curette involves scraping out the lining of the uterus (womb) through the vagina, under a general anaesthetic if you wish. The lining can then be examined under the microscope to see whether the bleeding was caused just by the oestrogens or by some other problem such as cancer of the lining of the uterus.

Men who take oestrogens also have their own special problems. These hormones can cause loss of interest in sex, impotence (inability to get an erection), decreased growth of facial hair, and enlargement of the breasts which can be painful. This last one can be prevented by giving the breast area a small dose of radiotherapy *before* starting your oestrogen treatment. Once it has developed, the only ways of getting rid of it are by stopping your oestrogen treatment or having your breasts removed surgically.

If you have unpleasant symptoms as a result of oestrogen treatments ask your doctors what the alternatives are. You may prefer a different form of hormone treatment or even to stop hormone treatment altogether.

Anti-Oestrogens

eg: tamoxifen

These drugs stop oestrogens from acting, they don't stop them from being produced. Anti-oestrogens can produce remissions of breast cancer in men or women of any age.

The dose of anti-oestrogen needed depends on how much oestrogen there is to be neutralised. This is why women who have active ovaries (women who are still having periods) need higher doses than women who don't have active ovaries (women who have passed the menopause either naturally or due to having their ovaries removed). These women do still have some oestrogens in their bodies because these hormones are also produced by the adrenal glands (and that's why men have some oestrogens in their bodies too).

Tamoxifen is a very good drug because most people taking it notice no side effects. Nafoxidine does however cause skin problems—rashes and excessive sensitivity to sunlight.

Any women taking anti-oestrogens may experience symptoms of menopause such as hot flushes, loss of interest in sex, a dry vagina, and irregularity or complete stopping of periods. These symptoms are more likely to trouble you if you have not yet passed your menopause.

Progesterone-Type Female Hormones

eg: medroxyprogesterone acetate (provera), megace

These hormones can produce remissions of cancer of the uterus and cancer of the breast. They can be taken either in tablet or injection form.

There are usually no side effects from progesterone-type treatments, but swelling of the ankles and weight gain can occur. If your uterus has not been removed, you will probably have bleeding similar to a period about two weeks after stopping your progesterone-type tablets. If you bleed at any other time, or if this bleeding is heavy or doesn't stop quickly by itself, you should consider having a curette (see page 283).

Male Hormones

eg: testosterone, nandrolone
    phenylpropionate

Male hormones can bring about remissions of breast cancer of women. They can stimulate the growth of prostate cancer and breast cancer in men so should be avoided by men who have these types of cancer. Male hormones are available both in tablet and injection form.

All women normally have small amounts of male hormone in their bodies. These are produced by the ovaries and the adrenal glands. Larger amounts are likely to cause deepening of the voice, growth of hair on the chin and upper lip, thinning of head hair, oiliness of the skin, and acne. The one which is likely to worry you the most is the growth of hair on the chin and upper lip. You could consider removing this regularly by depilatory creams, waxing or other methods. None of these side effects are permanent—they will all go back to normal once you stop taking the male hormones.

An uncommon side effect of male hormones is swelling of the ankles and weight gain due to passing too little salt and fluid out through the urine. Fluid tablets should correct this. Male hormones also occasionally cause yellow jaundice through bile building up in the liver. This can be quickly corrected by stopping the male hormone altogether or sometimes by changing to a different one.

If you are not prepared to put up with the side effects of male hormone, tell your doctor. It may be possible to switch to another one with less side effects or to try a completely different way of changing your hormone balance. Weigh up the various possibilities and decide what's best for you.

Corticosteroids

eg: prednisone, prednisolone, cortisone,
    hydrocortisone, dexamethasone

Corticosteroids are normally produced by our adrenal glands. As we have seen (page 281), they can help to produce remissions of acute lymphablastic leukaemia, chronic lymphocytic leukaemia, Hodgkin's disease, most non-Hodgkin's lymphomas and multiple myeloma. They can also produce remissions of breast cancer if taken in a dose that will inactivate your adrenal glands and so prevent them from producing sex hormones. Such a dose will also stop the adrenal glands from producing corticosteroids themselves.

Corticosteroids for Cancer Symptoms

In the types of cancer listed above, corticosteroids produce their benefits by acting against the cancer itself. Corticosteroids can also produce benefits in these and other types of cancer indirectly by acting on a complication of the cancer rather than the cancer itself. There are certain symptoms of cancer that can be controlled temporarily by corticosteroids, regardless of whether or not the cancer itself is sensitive to these hormones.

For example, corticosteroids can temporarily relieve the symptoms of cancer in the brain — headache, nausea and vomiting, drowsiness and blurred vision. They relieve these symptoms by reducing the swelling and pressure around the brain cancer, not by shrinking the cancer itself. By the same means, that is, reducing the swelling around it but not the size of the cancer itself, they can also temporarily improve breathing due to pressure on the wind pipe, congestion due to pressure on blood vessels, or numbness and paralysis of the legs due to pressure on the spinal cord.

Corticosteroids can also control symptoms of excessive calcium in the blood — nausea, vomiting, thirst and the production of very large amounts of urine. They do this simply by lowering the calcium level, not by acting on the cancer. They can also improve energy and appetite, again without having any effect on the cancer itself. Fever is another symptom that can be relieved by these hormones. Corticosteroids can also be used to treat a certain type of anaemia which is caused by some types of cancer. Anaemia due to antibodies against red blood cells (haemolytic anaemias) can often be corrected by corticosteroid treatment.

Side Effects of Corticosteroids

Whether corticosteroids are used to control symptoms, produce remissions or even to help permanently cure some cancers, their benefits come at a price. Corticosteroids have many side effects. They can be kept at a minimum by keeping the dose as low as possible and/or by taking them in short courses separated by breaks. Troublesome side effects are much more likely if you take them for more than a few weeks at a time in high doses.

I'll just explain here what I mean by a high dose. The daily dose that is about the same as your own adrenal glands would normally produce is about forty milligrams (mgs) of cortisone or about ten milligrams of prednisolone or prednisone or just over one milligram of dexamethasone. Anything more than these doses is a high dose and will make your own adrenal glands inactive if taken for more than two weeks at a stretch. Half or less of these doses is a low dose.

Corticosteroids come in tablet and injection forms. Fortunately almost none of their side effects are permanent. They will clear up sooner or later if you stop taking the corticosteroids.

The side effects which you are most likely to already know about are the changes in appearance that extra corticosteroids commonly produce. They cause weight gain but also change the location of fatty tissue so that you may develop a chubby face and trunk with loss of fat off the arms and legs. Your face may also look redder, and your skin generally may become thin and bruise easily or acne may develop.

The thinness in the arms and legs is due to loss of muscle as well as fat. After a few weeks or months on corticosteroid treatment you may notice muscle weakness, especially when climbing stairs, getting up from a squatting position or out of an easy chair.

While taking corticosteroids you may feel restless and bursting with energy, unusually emotional and excitable and have difficulty in sleeping. If these feelings are unpleasant, you could consider cutting down the dose of corticosteroids. Discuss this with your doctor.

Whether or not you have 'highs' on corticosteroids, you may feel flat, lacking in energy, depressed and weepy for some days after stopping them. This can be a serious problem if you are taking repeated short, high dose courses of corticosteroids. The withdrawal reaction can usually be prevented by cutting down your corticosteroid dose gradually over three or four days instead of stopping suddenly.

If you already have a tendency to sugar diabetes, corticosteroid treatment can bring this out. You could develop full-scale diabetes with excessive hunger and thirst and production of large amounts of urine. You may need insulin to get it under control. The diabetes would probably, but not definitely, disappear once you stopped taking the corticosteroids.

Extra corticosteroids interfere with fluid and mineral balance. While taking them, you will tend to retain fluid and salt—your ankles may swell and you may get short of breath, especially when lying down. This can be corrected with fluid tablets. You may also lose excessive amounts of potassium which can cause a general feeling of tiredness and muscle weakness. Ask your doctor to check the amount of potassium in your blood if you feel very lethargic. If it is low, it can be corrected by taking extra potassium in tablet form.

While taking corticosteroids, you will also have a lowered resistance to infections, especially those due to germs other than bacteria—thrush, for example (thrush is due to a fungus—see page 243). Any cuts, scratches or other wounds you have will not heal as well as they would normally. You should be sure to look after any wounds you have especially carefully. Keep them clean and protect them from further injury.

Extra corticosteroids can produce indigestion and heartburn, mainly through increasing acid in the stomach. Antacids will help these symptoms. It is quite dangerous to take corticosteroids if you have had stomach ulcers. They are likely to be aggravated and to bleed as a result.

High blood pressure can be caused or made worse by corticosteroids. Make sure your blood pressure is checked regularly while you are taking them.

If you take them for more than a few months, corticosteroids may weaken your bones. They will also stunt the growth of anyone who has not already reached their full height. This last one is a permanent effect.

Corticosteroid Deficiency

Our adrenal glands release a certain amount of corticosteroids into the blood under normal circumstances and very much more when we are under any serious stress, such as an operation, a serious infection or heavy bleeding. Symptoms of corticosteroid deficiency can occur whenever there are not enough of these hormones in our blood for the circumstances. Symptoms of corticosteroid deficiency include nausea, vomiting, diarrhoea, weakness and dizziness. Blood tests would show dehydration, low levels of sodium and high levels of potassium. Corticosteroid deficiency that is not corrected within just a few days is fatal.

It is extremely important that you understand that your adrenal glands will become completely inactive if you take high doses of corticosteroids for more than two weeks at a time. (In other words, if you are taking it in courses that are two weeks or less, or in low doses for longer periods, the following does *not* apply to you.)

As long as you take at least as much as your own glands would normally produce under all circumstances, you won't have any problems. You need to realise that your own glands will not produce any corticosteroids even when you are under stress—you will have to take extra artificially. You must also realise that they won't start working again immediately when you stop taking corticosteroids. In fact, it could take them some months to get back to normal.

Therefore you must make sure that you never run out of corticosteroid tablets or miss a dose for any reason. If you can't take a dose, say because of nausea and vomiting, contact your doctor and arrange to have it by injection. As soon as you are under any serious stress—such as an operation, a serious infection, or heavy bleeding, you must take very much higher doses of corticosteroids until you are well again. This is simply doing artificially what your own glands would normally do naturally.

If you have been taking a high dose of corticosteroids for more than two weeks, don't stop taking them suddenly. You will have to cut your dose down gradually, to give your adrenal glands a chance to recover. A complete recovery takes some months. To start with your adrenal glands may produce enough corticosteroids for normal day to day living but still be unable to produce extra under stress. You will need to take extra corticosteroids if you get, say, a serious infection or heavy bleeding, or have an operation within a few months of stopping long-term high-dose corticosteroid treatment.

Remember that symptoms of corticosteroid deficiency include nausea, vomiting, diarrhoea, weakness and dizziness. If you get these symptoms for no apparent reason while taking corticosteroids they could mean you are not taking enough. Check with your doctor immediately. There are blood tests that will tell whether or not your symptoms are due to a lack of corticosteroids.

If you take high dose corticosteroids for more than two weeks at a time you should wear a bracelet or carry a card at all times stating this. It is essential that, in case of any emergency, doctors know about your corticosteroid treatment.

You will have to weigh up the likely cost and benefits for yourself to decide whether or not to take corticosteroids in a particular situation. Keep in mind that you are unlikely to have any serious side effects or to run a risk of corticosteroid deficiency if you have treatment with them for only a few weeks at a time or in small doses for longer periods of time.

Aminoglutethimide

Aminoglutethimide is not a hormone but a chemical which stops the adrenal glands from producing hormones. It comes in tablet form. The adrenal glands are not permanently damaged by this drug. They will start producing hormones again normally within a few weeks of stopping aminoglutethimide treatment.

Aminoglutethimide can produce remissions of any cancers which are sensitive to male and/or female hormones (breast cancer of women of any age, breast and prostate cancers of men). It produces these remissions by stopping the adrenal glands from producing male and female hormones. However, this is not all it does — it also completely stops the adrenal glands from producing the corticosteroids we talked about on pages 286–90.

While you are taking aminoglutethimide, and for several weeks after you stop it, you must take as much corticosteroids as your adrenal glands would normally produce. If you don't do this you will get symptoms of corticosteroid deficiency and could even die. Read the last section to find out what the necessary doses of corticosteroids are, what the symptoms of deficiency of these hormones are, and how to avoid developing them. You would have to follow exactly the same precautions as a person who was taking high dose corticosteroids. You have to do artificially what your adrenal glands would normally do naturally.

It would also be important to wear a bracelet or carry a card at all times stating that you are taking aminoglutethimide. It would be essential for doctors to know this in any emergency.

Aminoglutethimide has other side effects besides those due to lack of corticosteroids. It can cause nausea, which can be reduced or prevented by gradually building up to a full dose over several weeks. Itchy, measles-like skin rashes are quite common in the first few weeks but will usually disappear even if you keep taking the aminoglutethimide. A vague lack of energy is sometimes a troublesome side effect of this drug, while a rare one is loss of balance.

Thyroid Hormone

eg: thyroxine, tri-iodothyronine
On pages 280–81, I explained a bit about the importance of taking

throxine if you have had a well differentiated cancer of the thyroid (papillary or follicular types).

The job of thyroid hormone is to keep the body functioning at a normal rate. If you have too little thyroid hormone in the blood, everything will work sluggishly. Symptoms can include lack of energy, unusual sensitivity to cold, depression, constipation, dry skin and weight gain in spite of a small appetite. If you have too much thyroid hormone in your blood, everything works too briskly. You could notice shakiness, unusual sweating, palpitations, irritability, difficulty sleeping, unusual sensitivity to heat, diarrhoea and weight loss in spite of a big appetite.

If you are taking thyroid hormone to prevent recurrence of thyroid cancer, you need to take enough to keep the amount in the blood slightly higher than normal. This will ensure that no cancer stimulating T.S.H. is released from the pituitary gland (see pages 280–81). You should not take so much that you get unpleasant symptoms of excessive thyroid hormone.

CHANGING THE HORMONE BALANCE BY REMOVING OR DESTROYING GLANDS
Removal Or Destruction Of The Ovaries (Oophorectomy)

Removal or destruction of the ovaries can produce remissions of breast cancer. This has a good chance of working only for women with active ovaries (women who have not yet reached the menopause). If it is more than eighteen months to two years since your last period, removal of your ovaries is unlikely to make enough difference to your hormone balance to produce a remission of your breast cancer. This is because your ovaries would be producing very little female hormone.

Removal of the ovaries can produce any of the symptoms which may occur during a normal menopause. These include hot flushes, mood swings, dryness of the vagina, loss of interest in sex, and, of course, no more periods. The last one's a certainty! These symptoms tend to be more severe after removal of the ovaries than during a normal menopause, because the amount of female hormone drops much more suddenly. Because the reason for removing the ovaries is to remove the source of female hormones, you would be completely defeating the purpose if you took female hormone for your symptoms of menopause.

Ask your doctor about the alternatives to removal of the ovaries. One is anti-oestrogen tablets (see page 284). These temporarily stop oestrogen-type female hormones from acting whereas surgery removes one of their sources permanently. Any symptoms of lack of female hormone will disappear whenever you stop taking anti-oestrogens. On the the other hand, once your ovaries have been removed, you're stuck with lack of female hormone, not just during the time (if any) while the treatment is acting against your cancer, but for the rest of your life.

Radiation of the ovaries is another alternative to removing them surgically. This can permanently stop your ovaries from working. You may prefer this to surgical removal if you don't feel physically or emotionally up to having an operation.

Removal Of The Testes (Orchidectomy)

Removal of the testes can produce remissions of prostate and breast cancer. This operation can result in decreased growth of facial hair, a higher voice, loss of interest in sex and loss of the ability to get an erection (impotence).

If you have prostate cancer, your main alternative is oestrogen treatment. I suggest you read pages 280 and 282–84.

If you have breast cancer, you have more alternatives. Read other relevant sections to help you to decide which is best for you.

Removal Of The Adrenal Glands

Removal of the adrenal glands can produce remissions of any cancer that is stimulated by either male or female hormones (breast cancer and prostate cancer). The adrenal glands are situated at the back of your abdominal cavity, just above each kidney. The idea of removing them is to remove an important source of male and female hormones but it is a very drastic way of doing this. Ask about all other alternatives before agreeing to it.

The problem is that this operation also permanently removes our *only* source of corticosteroid homones. As we have seen, these hormones are essential for life (see pages 289–90). If your adrenal glands are removed, you must take as much corticosteroids as they would normally have produced, for the rest of your life. This means taking about forty milligrams (mg) of cortisone or ten milligrams of prednisone or one to one-and-a-half milligrams of dexamethasone every day and much more whenever you are under stress. Read pages 289–90 which explain the importance of taking your corticosteroids correctly, the symptoms of corti-costeroid deficiency and what to do to prevent these from happening.

If your adrenals are removed, you should at all times carry a card or wear a bracelet stating this. It is essential that, in any emergency, your doctors know that you must be given large amounts of corticosteroids.

What are the alternatives to removal of your adrenal glands? With breast cancer, the chance of this operation producing a remission is similar to the many other ways of favourably changing the hormone balance. Remember that there is even another way of stopping your adrenals from producing hormones. Aminoglute-thimide (see pages 290–91) can do this by chemical means and has the major advantage of producing only a temporary effect. Whenever the treatment is not controlling your cancer, it can be stopped and your adrenal glands will start working normally again within a few weeks. If they've been removed, you're stuck with taking replacement hormones, not just for the time (if any) during which the treatment is working against your cancer, but for the rest of your life.

Removal Or Destruction Of The Pituitary Gland

Removal or destruction of the pituitary gland is sometimes recommended for the treatment of cancers whose growth is likely to be stimulated by male or female hormones. It is a very drastic way of changing the balance of sex hormones and a method that I would never agree to for myself.

Your pituitary gland is inside your skull bone just behind your eyes and above and behind your nose. The pituitary can actually be removed only by a major operation through the outside of the skull. It is easier to destroy it, by putting ice cold probes or radioactive substances or alcohol into it via the nose.

The pituitary gland controls the thyroid gland, and adrenal glands as well as the ovaries and testes. It also produces some hormones of its own, including one which helps to control the mineral and water balance (anti-diuretic hormone or A.D.H. for short).

Without a pituitary gland, all of the glands which are controlled by it become inactive. Therefore, if your pituitary gland is removed or destroyed, you would have to take thyroid hormone and corticosteroids for the rest of your life. You would have all the symptoms of lack of male or female hormones. You would also be likely to suffer from lack of A.D.H., the main symptom of which is passing very large amounts of very watery urine. Replacement A.D.H. cannot be taken in tablet form but only as injections or as a spray or powder squirted into the nose.

If your pituitary gland is removed or destroyed, you must carry a card or wear a bracelet stating this at all times. It is essential that any doctors treating you in an emergency know that you need all the hormones normally controlled by the pituitary gland.

CONCLUSION

This book is about making choices— creative, responsible, positive choices. It is about not giving in passively to anything— to your cancer, to your doctors, to your treatment or to your symptoms. It is about recognising and accepting that *you* are the greatest possible expert on yourself. It is about knowing that there are always choices and that there is *never* anything that you *have* to do. It is about looking for those choices, finding out about each one, and combining that information with your own unique knowledge of yourself to come up with the decision that is best for you. It is about being flexible and kind to yourself.

I have not given you any easy solutions in this book, because I don't believe there are any. There is no one course of action that is right for everyone. There are no all-knowing experts who will always make exactly the right decisions on your behalf. I'm afraid life just isn't that easy.

If you try to follow the advice I have given you in this book, you may go through some very difficult times when you doubt your own judgement because the pressures on you are so great. Keep trusting yourself— you *do* know what's best.

Here is a thought that might help during those hard times. Every time you demand more information, refuse to accept instructions willy-nilly, and insist on making your own decisions, you make it just that bit easier for the people coming after you. Doctors are not used to being questioned or to having their advice rejected and some of them handle these experiences like spoilt children. Stand firm— they need to learn that patients are people, people with minds of their own who are perfectly capable of making their own decisions provided they get the necessary information. Doctors *will* change their attitudes if they are confronted by enough people often enough.

Well, here's hoping you succeed in making the very best possible of the rest of your life, however long or short that may be! If you've been brave enough to read this book, I know you've got what it takes. Go for it!

USEFUL ADDRESSES

British Association of Cancer United Patients
(BACUP)
121-3 Charterhouse Street
London EC1M 6AA
Tel: 01 608 1785/6
(An information service contactable in office hours to help cancer sufferers, and their friends and families, to understand more about the illness, and to provide practical advice on how to cope.)

Cancer Aftercare and Rehabilitation Society
Lodge Cottage
Church Lane
Timsbury
Bath BA3 1LF
Tel: 0761 70731

Cancer Contact
Honorary Organiser: 0444 454043
Honorary Treasurer and Support Section: 0444 413055

Cancer Help Centre
Grove House
Cornwallis Grove
Clifton
Bristol BS8 4PG
Tel: 0272 743216

Cancer Prevention Society
25 Wellington Street
Glasgow
Tel: 041 226 4626

CancerLink
46 Pentonville Road
London N1 9HF
Tel: 01 833 2451
(A support and information service for people with cancer and their families. Instigates the formation of support groups, and can provide a directory of all existing support groups on request.)

Compassionate Friends
5 Lower Clifton Hill
Clifton
Bristol
Tel: 0272 292778
(Can put bereaved parents in touch with self-help groups and counsellors.)

CRUSE
Cruse House
126 Sheen Road
Richmond
Surrey TW9 1UR
(Local branches can offer support and advice to widows, widowers and their children.)

Friends of Shanti Nilaya
Old Cherry Orchard
Forest Row
East Sussex
(Shanti Nilaya is Sanskrit for 'home of peace', and is the name of the centre established by Dr Elizabeth Kubler Ross in California, where she holds workshops for people who are dying or bereaved in

order to help them come to terms with grief. Friends of Shanti Nilaya carries out similar support work in England.)

Help the Hospices
BMA House
Tavistock Square
London WC1H 9JP
Tel: 01 388 7807
(Acts as a national voice for the hospice movement and raises funds at a national level, mainly for training and education, to spread hospice expertise. Also grants money for hospice projects.)

Hospice Information Service
St Christopher's Hospice
Lawrie Park Road
London SE26 6DZ
Tel: 01 778 1240/9252
(Provides information about hospice-style care available in Britain and Eire. A full directory is available on receipt of a large s.a.e.)

Hysterectomy Support Group
Rivendell
Warren Way
Lower Heswall
Wirral
Merseyside
Tel: 051 342 3167
or 11 Henryson Road
London SE4 1HL

Leukaemia Care Society
PO Box 82
Exeter
Devon EX2 5LP
Tel: 0592 218514

The Marie Curie Memorial Foundation
28 Belgrave Square
London SW1X 8OQ
Tel: 01 235 3325
(A national charity which runs homes providing care for the dying, and which offers nursing services for the dying in local communities.)

Mastectomy Association
26 Harrison Street
off Gray's Inn Road
King's Cross
London WC1H 8JG
Tel: 01 837 0908

NAC (New Approaches to Cancer)
c/o The Seekers Trust
The Close
Addington Park
Near Maidstone
Kent ME19 5BL
Tel: 0732 848336

National Society for Cancer Relief
15-19 Britten Street
London SW3 3TY
Tel: 01 351 7811
(Provides financial assistance for patients and relatives in need through its Patient Grants Department. Applications should be made by local authority, hospital or hospice social workers. The society also funds home care [Macmillan] nurses in the community and in National Health Service hospitals.)

Sue Ryder Foundation
Sue Ryder Home
Cavendish
Suffolk CO10 8AY
Tel: 09787 280252
(A national charity which runs a number of homes, including
several for people with advanced cancer.)

Women's National Cancer Control Campaign
1 South Audley Street
London W1Y 5DQ
Tel: 01 499 7532/4

INDEX